Alaska's Search for a Killer

Alaska's Search for a Killer

A Seafaring Medical Adventure
1946 to 1948

Susan Meredith
with Kitty Gair and Elaine Schwinge

Alaska Public Health Nursing History Association

Meredith, Susan H.
  Alaska's Search for a Killer
  A Seafaring Medical Adventure, 1946-1948
  Published by Alaska Public Health Nursing History Association
  Juneau, Alaska
  Copyright 1998 by Susan Meredith

Permission is given by Will Nordby to reprint kayaking portions of the manuscript originally published as "Alaskan Remembrances" in his anthology, *Seekers of the Horizon*. Chester, Connecticut; The Globe Pequot Press, 1989.

Editor: Lorna Price
Book design and cover: Jean Meredith

Pictures from Susan Meredith's collection with contributions from Territory of Alaska Department of Health files, Kitty Gair, Elaine Schwinge, Forrest Bates, Peggy MacNair, and Ronald Heilman.

Publisher's Cataloging-in-Publication Data
(Provided by Quality Books Inc.)

Meredith, Susan H.
  Alaska's search for a killer: a seafaring medical adventure,
  1946-1948 / Susan H. Meredith. – – 1st. ed.
    p. cm.
  Includes bibliographical references.
  ISBN 0-9659849-1-5

  1. Tuberculosis—Alaska. 2. Alaska—History—1867-1959. I. Title.

RA644.T7M47 1997   614.5'42'09798
                               QB197-41011

Printed in the United States of America

To my mother, who encouraged me to pursue my dreams
and who saved my letters,

and

To Kitty Gair and Elaine Schwinge, M.D., my friends and shipmates,
who symbolize the many dedicated nurses and doctors who over the years
left the comforts of their contemporary world to bring a modern medical
program to the far-flung villages of the Territory of Alaska.

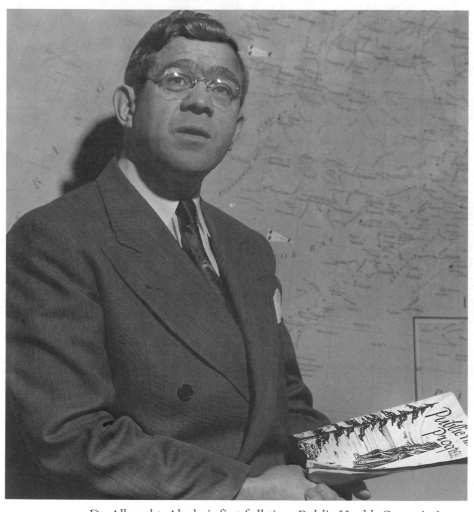

Dr. Albrecht, Alaska's first full-time Public Health Commissioner

Preface

EVIDENCE SUGGESTS that the early fur traders brought diseases to the susceptible Native populations of Alaska from the rest of the world. These people had no natural immunity: smallpox, measles, whooping cough, and influenza decimated the Native population. Tuberculosis and venereal diseases ran rampant in overcrowded living quarters. Before that time the Native population was mainly concerned with finding enough food and surviving injuries received in occasional battles.

After the U.S. bought Alaska in 1867, it became a "forgotten land," with no representation and no power to enact laws or levy taxes until 1884, when Congress established Alaska's first civil government. In 1903, a long-standing boundary dispute between the U.S. and Canada over the Alaska Panhandle was settled, and it resulted in a period of rapid building and development in Alaska. The Territory of Alaska was created in 1912.

One of Alaska's early physicians, Dr. H.C. DeVigne, described in his book, *Time of My Life,* conditions he found in the early 1900s. He wrote:

> The only law in Alaska applicable to the healing art, enacted for the Territory by an indifferent Congress, but not even indifferently enforced, provided that to procure a license to treat the sick one must possess a diploma from a medical school and pay a five dollar recording fee. No one bothered to inquire whether the degree was from a reputable institution or whether it had been earned, bought or stolen or in fact whether or not it was a medical diploma.

During the gold rush days, individual towns set up their own rules and regulations for burying the dead and isolating the sick. In 1913 the first appointed governor of Alaska was named Commissioner of Health by the newly formed Territorial Legislature. After six years the Territorial Legislature created the office of Commissioner of Health and appointed a physician to head it on a part-time basis. Three part-time divisional representatives and a part-time stenographer assisted him. This structure continued until 1936.

Passage of the Social Security Act in 1936 provided federal funding and marked the expansion of staff and services and the beginning of public health activities in Alaska. Unsuccessful attempts were made in the 1939 and 1941 sessions of the Territorial Legislature to pass an act legalizing the Territorial Department of Health.

After the declaration of war in 1941, Alaska became a strategic area. Draft records indicated a high incidence of disease in the Native population and a great need for public health services. But at this time few people were available to deliver them; during the war, public health programs in Alaska were reduced to emergency measures.

In 1945 the Territorial Legislature of Alaska legalized the Health Department and created the first territory-wide Board of Health. They selected and employed Dr. C. Earl Albrecht to be the first full-time Commissioner of Health. He proved to be an excellent choice. In a few months he worked with Governor Ernest Gruening to call a special session of the Territorial Legislature. There he persuaded the lawmakers to increase their appropriation of funds to fight TB from $30,000 to $250,000, one tenth of the Territory's annual budget.

Alaska's extremes in size, geography, climate, and cultures challenged the newly created Health Department to develop some innovative and expensive programs to reach its widely scattered population. To meet this challenge, the department was acquiring mobile units to be transported by plane, train, truck, and ship.

A team of physicians from the American Medical Association reported that tuberculosis was the most urgent health problem in Alaska. It was listed as the cause of death on 43 percent of all death certificates for Alaska Natives. The overall death rate was nearly nine times that of the rest of the U.S. With this information, Dr. Albrecht and Governor Gruening convinced the 80th U.S. Congress to make available surplus World War II ships and military hospitals in Alaska, and also personnel to provide mobile health services. This enabled the Territorial Department of Health to field one solution, among others, to the problem—a floating health clinic named the MV *Hygiene*.

Dr. Albrecht and the Board of Health hoped the *Hygiene* would be a major factor in solving the apparent epidemic of tuberculosis in Alaska. At that time, treatment consisted of months or years of bed rest in a sanitarium, and occasionally thoracic surgery. Statistics on the number of victims of this dreaded disease, and where they were located, were essential in order to determine where to build hospitals.

The *Hygiene's* primary mission was to screen the entire coastal population for tuberculosis. We were to identify other serious medical problems that appeared and treat them when possible. It seemed a straightforward, clear-cut task.

During the MV *Hygiene's* first innovative voyages, our medical staff and crew found challenge, kinship, and cooperation, as well as occasional conflict in the course of our odyssey through Alaska's remote and sometimes hostile waters. This is our story as well as the story of many memorable, resourceful, and adventurous residents of the communities we visited.

Acknowledgments

A very special thank you to Kitty Gair and Elaine Schwinge for their help and support throughout this project; for their reports, diaries, excerpts from letters, pictures and memories, and for help in writing and checking the accuracy of the text.

I appreciate the support of Dr. and Mrs. C. Earl Albrecht for their interest and help. I am grateful to Neil and Rosemarie Davis who encouraged me to put this material together in the form of a book and have helped me through the complexities of writing and publishing, and to Lee Sturdivant for her advice in the field of self-publishing. And I thank Carla Helfferick and Ellen Wheat who gave me editorial advice. I am further indebted to Walter VomLehn, Mike Kaill, and Joan Schwinge, who read the manuscript for clarity and accuracy. I also thank Vivian Landbeck, Nell Hales, George and Marietta Koch, Dawn Anderson, Sam Connery, Trudy and John Dallas, Susan Harris, Robin Donnelly, Shirley and Tom Alvis, Sally Webb, and Linda Badten. I want to thank Chuck Boatman, George Yount, Tom Linder, and Jim Slocomb, who helped me enter the world of computers and who fixed problems that arose. Much appreciated was the help from the librarians of the Friday Harbor Library and from Griffin Bay Bookstore.

Special thanks go to Lorna Price, my editor and friend, to Jean Meredith, my daughter and book designer, to Louise Dustrude, my proof reader, and to Wolfgang Chamberlain, who drew the deck plans of the *Hygiene*, and to Jim, my husband, who supplied words I needed and put up with my periodic retreats to that other world in Alaska.

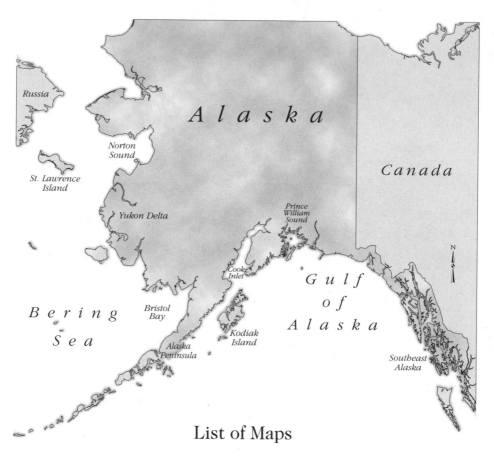

List of Maps

Table of Contents

Introduction

Seattle 1975

ANOTHER RAINY DAY, another compulsion to clean the cobwebbed corners of our basement. With a sigh, I opened a dusty trunk that had moldered there since my mother's death 20 years earlier. The first bundle I pulled out consisted of a large stack of handwritten letters held together with dried-out rubber bands. They proved to be letters I had written to my invalid mother between 1946 and 1948 when I had worked in Alaska as a bacteriologist and X-ray technician on the Public Health Ship MV *Hygiene*.

I started to read a paragraph here and there. Soon I was transported back to the wild coastline of Alaska. No longer was I a housewife and a mother involved in PTA, Girl Scouts, grocery shopping, and gardening. My mind skipped the 25 intervening years, and I was back on board the ship that I had lived on and loved. Again I saw the Natives in their fur-trimmed parkas gathered on the beach of a Bering Sea village, waiting to welcome us. Again I felt the total exhaustion of working 16-hour days when the weather was good, and enduring the swells and banging from side to side in my bunk when it wasn't. Again I empathized with the joy of a toothless, grinning Eskimo granny as she waved her X-ray card marked "negative for TB."

I realized these letters were a tiny but important focus on part of Alaska's history. They described the first two years of a generalized mobile public health program for coastal Alaska—the only all-territorial organized health care program since the Russians had sold that vast land to the United States. Dedicated doctors, nurses, teachers, and priests had traveled to many isolated areas of Alaska, but no system had been devised to reach all of the far-flung, widely separated villages so desperately in need of help.

I recalled an earlier letter I had written to Alaska's Territorial Department of Health in Juneau just after World War II ended, asking if they had any openings for a bacteriologist in a coastal town. Frustrations of working at a necessary but routine hospital job in Seattle during World War II had prompted my query.

After an anxious two weeks, I received a letter from Alaska's Department of Health, Division of Laboratories. In disappointment, I read that no positions were available in their laboratories. But as I continued reading, I could not believe my eyes: the Health Department was putting a public health mobile unit into service on a ship, and they would need a bacteriologist and X-ray technician. Would I be interested?

Would I?

I had contracted polio as a child and spent many months in plaster casts. In those periods of forced inactivity, I read adventure books by the score, dreaming alternately of being a cowgirl or a sailor. Now was my chance to try one of these roles in real life.

After earning a degree in bacteriology I had worked in the State of Washington Public Health Laboratory and the U.S. Army's 9th Service Command Laboratory as well as a hospital lab, but I knew nothing about taking X-rays. The hospital X-ray department was across the hall from the lab where I worked, so I asked the technicians if it would be possible to learn what I would need to know about X-raying in three months. They were certain that with my background I could. With that encouragement, I immediately accepted the job in Alaska, telling them I would brush up on my X-ray techniques.

Shortly after that Mr. Martinson, the General Electric sales representative responsible for installing the X-ray machine on the *Hygiene*, contacted me. He led me into the world of X-ray, making it possible for me to get maximum experience in a short time. He had an ulterior motive: he wanted his machine to be cared for properly.

For three months I lived and breathed X-ray. I spent as much time as I could in the hospital learning general X-ray techniques. I worked as a volunteer on a State of Washington mobile X-ray truck for two months, learning to use the same type of machine I would have on the ship. Classes on the mechanics and electrical circuits of X-ray machines occupied my evenings— where we were going, there would be no repairmen.

The following account is derived from information in the letters I wrote to my mother, from my diary and reports, from Kitty Smulling Gair's letters and nursing reports, from Dr. Elaine Schwinge's diary and medical reports, and from copies of other medical reports that Kitty kept. Statistics are at a minimum, because unfortunately the official records of the Alaska Department of Health for the first six months of this period were stored in a garage and destroyed when the garage burned. Those figures that we quote are from our personal files.

In addition to describing in detail the public health mission of the *Hygiene* and its diverse crew, I hope to convey a sense of the majestic natural beauty of Alaska as well as the rigorous daily existence of its people.

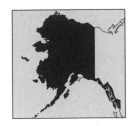

1

Seattle to Juneau

1946

The forerunner of the Hygiene, *the little* Hy-Gene, *a smaller ship, had proved that the concept of a marine clinic was feasible. However, a larger and more seaworthy vessel was needed to cross the Gulf of Alaska. Moored alongside the larger ship, the little* Hy-Gene *served as temporary quarters for the skeleton crew.*

Lake Union Dry Dock
Monday, April 15, to Wednesday, May 15, 1946

MY STOMACH WAS CHURNING as I searched the docks at Lake Union ship yard, anxiously looking for the MV *Hygiene.* Then I saw her looming above the throngs of fishing boats undergoing repairs for the coming season. Workmen swarmed over her, and the noise of their pounding hammers and machinery was deafening. Timidly I threaded my way through a jumble of exposed bulkhead frames, wires, and lumber and asked for Captain Darrell Naish. A tall, blond man in his thirties stepped forward and greeted me warmly, saying, "We've been expecting you. Come on into the galley where we can talk above the din. The rest of the crew is in there having a mug-up (coffee break)."

As we made our way along the littered deck he explained that the ship-yard crew were transforming the cargo hold of the 114-foot former army freight-supply ship—a seaworthy vessel that had served in the Aleutians—into a public health clinic that would consist of a doctor's and a nurse's

5

office, an examining room, laboratory, and a modern General Electric X-ray machine and darkroom. Above were a secretary's office, a waiting room, and heads (bathrooms). Later a small dental office was added. The remainder of the vessel was given over to the engine room, a galley, dining salon, and crew and medical staff quarters.

Darrell introduced me to the trio sitting around the galley table. I was apprehensive, but eager to meet Kitty Smulling, the nurse. We would be working closely together. Gus Gair, the chief engineer, a tall, angular man with a deadpan face that looked as though it would crack if he smiled, and Rex Fox, the mate, were rather quiet at first. Then Rex, a shorter, rounder man with mischievous eyes, asked, "Do you have a car? We should have some fun while we're here." I offered to drive them wherever they wanted to go in my rattling Model A Ford. Rex, looking completely serious, suggested, "Why don't we go downtown and get a hotel room?" Gus joined in, "That sounds like a good idea."

I had led a sheltered life and did not know how to handle this remark. I wondered what kind of a situation I was getting into. Kitty, seeing my confusion, quickly said, "It's dinner time—why don't we all go to that Italian restaurant nearby and get better acquainted?" As she and I lagged behind the men, she chuckled, explaining, "You've undergone a test these crew members give to all female newcomers. Just don't believe anything they say." I liked Kitty right away, and we soon became allies against the teasing of Gus and Rex.

Kitty, who had been on board for two weeks, worried about her lack of knowledge of marine matters. Born in Pennsylvania, she had little experience with the sea. "I once rowed a half mile on the Juniata River, spent a weekend yachting on Chesapeake Bay, and I did travel to Alaska on the *Northland* three years ago. But I can never remember which side is port and which is starboard and I keep forgetting to call the front the bow and the back the stern, and what's worse I can't seem to remember to lift my feet high enough to clear these high door-sills." She showed me a row of bruises on her shins.

But she was an experienced public health nurse and had previously worked for the Territory in Anchorage. She described a little of what might lie ahead. Our primary mission was to search for cases of tuberculosis—to gather statistics on the coastal population of Alaska from Nome to the Canadian border. We would use X-rays, laboratory tests, and physical examinations to determine both the extent of TB and the places where it was most prevalent. We would treat other serious medical problems when possible.

I had worked in public health laboratories, but I was not familiar with the nursing philosophy of public health. Kitty explained, "As a public health nurse, my primary focus is to educate people to keep themselves well." Kitty worried because she would have to do a fair amount of clinical nursing that would limit her teaching and counseling time. These considerations did not bother me, since my job was clearcut—or so I thought.

I lived in Seattle and wouldn't move aboard until the ship left. Through visits, however, I became better acquainted with and less intimidated by my future shipmates.

Darrell was calm and easygoing, and had a good sense of humor. Gus, the engineer, and Rex, the mate, had grown up and gone to school together in Douglas, Alaska, and though they had gone different ways during the war, they were again a team and teased Kitty and me unmercifully. I felt a great deal of sympathy for the little girls who had once been their schoolmates. Johnny Camp, the 2nd engineer, seemed eager to put off till tomorrow whatever he could, and George, just out of high school, was the deckhand.

Seattle to Juneau
Thursday, May 16, to Sunday, May 19

May 16, the day of our departure, dawned bright and clear. Despite the unfinished carpentry, the unpainted clinic, and the jumble of medical supplies, we sailed for Juneau. Friends had said their last good-byes. Dr. Albrecht, Alaska's first full-time Commissioner of Health and the driving force behind the *Hygiene's* program, joined us for the trip north. He was so excited the night before we left, he shook hands with all the departing visitors, even bidding a mistaken farewell to Gus, our chief engineer.

We sailed through the Ballard locks into Puget Sound and dense fog. Our foghorn responded to several other deep-throated horns as we crawled along for three hours. Then a minor catastrophe occurred. I slipped on some fuel left on the deck when the tanks were filled and slammed my great toe against the bulwarks. I felt excruciating pain and heard the bone crack! It was evident that my toe was dislocated. Kitty and Dr. Albrecht searched through the boxes of medical supplies for some Novocain. Dr. Albrecht also needed an X-ray to determine if the bone might be fractured as well as dislocated. I commented, "It's lucky it wasn't my head, or there would be no one to tell you how to use the X-ray machine." Sure enough, a bone chip was lodged in the joint, preventing it from going back into place. From the height of excitement I quickly fell

Main Deck

Winches

Fo'c'sle ladder

Secretary's office

Dentist's office

Waiting room

Stairs to clinic

Patients head

Patient's head

Susie's stateroom
closet
bench
bunk
wash basin

Dentist's stateroom

Gus's stateroom

Kitty's stateroom

Men's head

Women's head

Ladder to engine room

Stairs to bridge

Galley

Dining salon

table

Stairs to
staterooms below
Doctor, Secretary,
and Cook

Generator

These are conceptual
drawings based on a 50
year old memory. They
are *not* to scale.

Upper Deck and Bridge

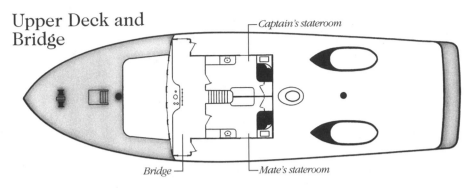

Captain's stateroom

Bridge

Mate's stateroom

Lower Deck

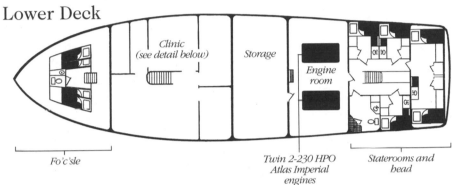

Clinic (see detail below)

Storage

Engine room

Fo'c'sle

Twin 2-230 HPO Atlas Imperial engines

Staterooms and head

Detail of Clinic

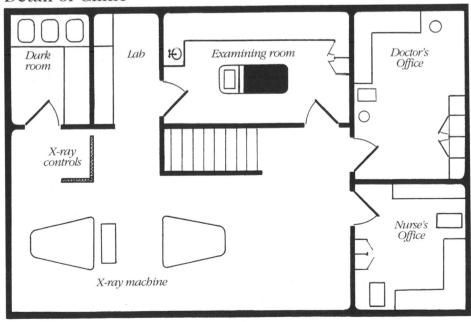

Dark room

Lab

Examining room

Doctor's Office

X-ray controls

Nurse's Office

X-ray machine

into the depths of despair. While Gus unlashed the X-ray machine, he teased. "Just couldn't wait to use your new machine, could you?"

Soon the fog lifted, the sun came out, and the *Hygiene* resumed her normal cruising speed of 10 knots, passing through the San Juan Islands and up the Strait of Georgia to the north end of Vancouver Island. Mountains towered to the west, and low-lying forested islands lay in front of another spectacular range to the east. On our second day, we crossed the unprotected waters of Queen Charlotte Sound and rolled and pitched for four hours until we entered the Inside Passage.

During this time I worried about what would happen to me. I was unable to walk on my heel, due to the polio I had contracted as a child, so now I was somewhat immobile. I was afraid I would be fired because of this handicap. My depression evaporated when Dr. Albrecht assured me that I would be able to continue this job of my dreams—the fall, due to an oversight of the deck crew, could have happened to anyone on board. Later I found some crew members were worried I would sue them. Dr. Albrecht was most sympathetic and planned to send me to the hospital in Juneau where they could surgically repair my toe. He thought I would probably be able to work by the time the ship was ready to leave.

On our third day we entered the 21-mile length of Wrangell Narrows, a beautiful but dangerously narrow and shallow passage. Darrell was carefully making his way along the well-marked channel when suddenly we lurched. We had struck bottom! A red marker buoy had caught fire and burned black, and Darrell had taken it on the wrong side. Fortunately the ship was not noticeably damaged, but Gus suffered a severe cut on his forehead, requiring seven stitches, when the jolt threw him against the engine room ladder. Four memorable days after we left Seattle, we arrived in Juneau, our home port and headquarters of the Alaska Territorial Department of Health.

Juneau
Monday, May 20, to Sunday, June 2

Dr. Albrecht immediately sent me to the hospital for surgery on my toe. I will never forget the kindness of the people in the health department to a total stranger. A steady stream of visitors brought books and candy and offered me transportation.

For two weeks the *Hygiene's* crew completed projects in preparation for our first working trip. The engineers installed the ventilation system in the clinic.

The cook and medical staff procured and stored our final supplies, while numerous visitors—ordinary citizens, doctors, and visiting health department staff members—flowed through the new ship, the pride of Alaska.

Dr. Berneta Block moved on board to be the ship's physician for the next six weeks. She proved to be the ideal choice. She had worked on the little *Hy-Gene*, and earlier had served 10 years in Korea as a medical missionary. This gentle lady constantly had us looking for lost birds as she practiced her hobby of imitating the songs and chirps of wild birds.

The clerk, Clarabelle Messerschmidt, an imposing peroxide blonde, had come aboard with preconceived ideas of what she would and would not do. She soon learned that working on board a ship was a team effort, and in a very short time she proved to be a hard worker and a good shipmate.

When the Army ran the *Hygiene* she had had a crew of 18 to 20 men. Darrell replaced the second engineer and deckhand and now with the addition of Helen, the cook, and a mess boy, Tommy, age 16 our crew numbered seven. Deckhand Forrest Bates, recently retired from a lonely Coast Guard station, proved himself useful to both the crew and the medical staff.

Released from the hospital after four days, I came back aboard on crutches under orders to keep my foot elevated. Unfortunately the wound had become infected. What a way to start! I was determined to carry on, but Kitty and Dr. Block scolded me whenever I moved off my bunk. Forrest, who was interested in photography and had experience developing film, was assigned the job of helping me with X-raying until I was more ambulatory. I had plenty of time to check and recheck my list of supplies as I lay on my bunk, but I was frustrated at not being able to see them and having to depend on others to fit everything into the crowded quarters, and yet I was so grateful that they could do it.

Finally everything was almost ready, and the *Hygiene* left Juneau, bound for Angoon. Carpentry and painting were still unfinished, but Dr. Albrecht thought it was wisest that we make a trial run first.

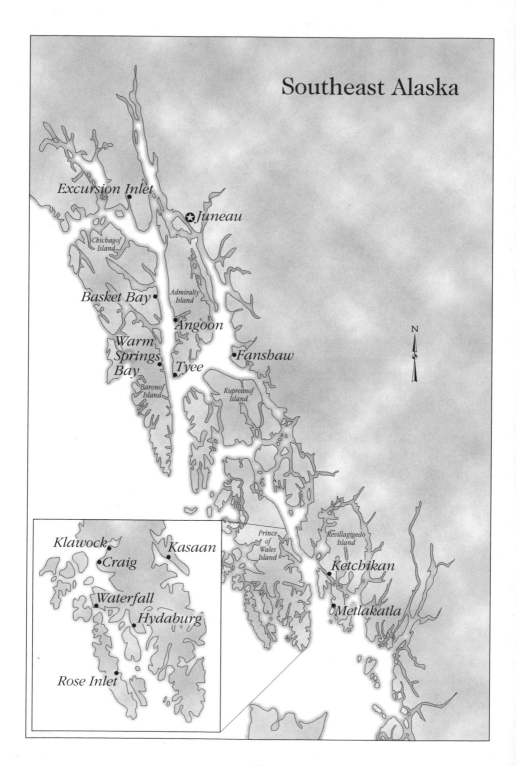

Southeast Alaska

Excursion Inlet

Juneau

Chichagof
Island

Basket Bay

Admiralty
Island

Angoon

Warm
Springs
Bay

Tyee

Fanshaw

Baronof
Island

Kupreanof
Island

Klawock

Craig

Kasaan

Waterfall

Hydaburg

Prince
of
Wales
Island

Revillagigedo
Island

Ketchikan

Metlakatla

Rose Inlet

N

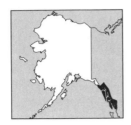

2

Southeast Alaska: Trial Run

Southeast Alaska's many sheltering islands protect its waters, although fog, rain, strong winds, tide rips, and reefs complicate navigation. In general the population of this region consisted mainly of Indians in the villages and whites in the larger towns. Most of the Natives spoke English. Some medical care was available. They were able to travel to doctors or hospitals by mail boat, fishing boat, or even plane if necessary and they could afford it.

Angoon
Monday, June 3, to Friday, June 7

Dr. Block, Kitty, Clarabelle, and I sat around the galley table as we traveled the 80 miles down Chatham Strait to our first assignment. Outside, rain pelted down from gray skies, but the galley was warm and filled with the odor of a roast in the oven. We reviewed our plans to the last detail.

Dr. Block assured us that the teachers and village leaders would be ready for us because the Juneau office planned to notify each village of our time of arrival. Then she went over the duty roster. "Clarabelle, you will get the census as soon as the ship arrives, and you can fill out the X-ray cards. Susie, if you have any time left after setting up for the X-rays, you can help Clarabelle with the cards. Kitty, you and I will go ashore immediately and schedule the people to arrive for their X-rays at a comfortable rate. By the time you have completed the survey X-rays, Susie, I will have a chance to look over the wet films and note any obvious abnormalities. If any show up, you can take full size X-rays on those cases while Kitty and I are doing the physical exams. That way we can complete the work on the patients before they leave the ship." It all sounded very efficient.

Angoon, a typical Southeast Alaska Native village of about 200 inhabitants, was located on a point. The water on one side was exposed to the wind and waves; the other was a narrow channel protected from wind, but subject to extreme tidal currents. The town had no dock. Because the weather! Forecast was good Darrell anchored in a bay a quarter-mile off the exposed shore, and we waited for someone to come out. While we waited, we took pictures of our first Indian community. Single-family dwellings mixed with wooden double-storied tribal houses formed uneven lines along the beach and stilted boardwalk.

A dark evergreen forest hovered over this small village. The schoolhouse was a frame building exactly like many in the States and three churches were prominent in the view. We later learned they were Presbyterian, Russian Orthodox, and Salvation Army, and that two stores supplied the people's needs.

An hour passed, and no one came to the ship, so Rex ferried Dr. Block and Kitty ashore in our small outboard to find the village teachers and get the census. The surprised teachers apologized; they had no idea we were coming. This was the first departure from our schedule. Soon our carefully laid plans were in a shambles.

Early the next morning Dr. Block and Kitty went ashore and found the town streets deserted. Long hours of daylight kept people up late, and they slept late in the morning—an old Alaska custom, we were told. We became aware that we had much to learn about Native culture and history. When the villagers finally came to the ship for their X-rays, confusion reigned. Clarabelle tried to put families together by name as they came in. She did not know children were often the responsibility of the maternal uncle and went by his name.

The narrow stairway to the clinic proved a problem, because it was only wide enough for one-way traffic. Part of a family would be above and the rest below. Children cried loudly when they could not find or get to their parents.

Rex ferried villagers and staff back and forth until the outboard died, leaving him with a boatload of Natives halfway between shore and the *Hygiene*. Much to his embarrassment, an older Indian woman looked at the silent motor, made a few adjustments, and brought it back to life. After that Rex turned the ferrying over to the villagers.

At dinner on June 5, after two days of nonstop crises, Kitty said to Dr. Block, "I don't know how you do it. Nothing seems to fluster you."

Dr. Block, in her gentle way, reminded Kitty, "I have the advantage of the rest of you, remember; I worked on the little *Hy-Gene*, and it was much smaller and less well equipped than this boat. You just can't expect things to go as they would ashore."

Just then Darrell came down from the pilot house, where he had been listening for radio messages supposed to be broadcast to us at 5:30 p.m. each day. Laughing, he said, "Well, that explains why they didn't know we were coming."

"Why?" we questioned.

"I just got a call from the Alaska Communications System asking anyone in the area of Angoon to relay a message to the Angoon operator—they can't raise him. The message—'The *Hygiene* will be arriving June 3.'"

"No wonder they were surprised," chuckled Dr. Block. "Well, so much for depending on the radio. And mail service isn't much better," she went on to console us.

Once they understood our schedule, the Indians were eager to obtain our services. They knew they needed medical care, and tuberculosis was a disease they greatly feared. The whirring sound of the X-ray machine frightened a few people, but when I told them I was just taking their picture, they were reassured and even smiled and "looked pretty" for the camera.

Dr. Block gave physical exams to all the children and to the adults who had health problems. Kitty weighed, measured, and vision-tested each child. She gave immunization shots to those who needed them and brought their records up to date. This was one area of health care that had not been as badly neglected as others. Henry Clark in his *History of Alaska* explains:

> Around 1836 the Russian America Company at Sitka had smallpox vaccine and tried to vaccinate the Natives. They refused because they had greater faith in the power of their shamans than in the Russians' medicine. But when approximately one quarter of the Native population died during an epidemic, and not a single vaccinated Russian was lost, the Natives came from great distances and in large numbers to be vaccinated, convinced of the merits of Russian medicine. The first U.S. nurses and doctors to appear in Alaska after the purchase from the Russians found the Natives eager for vaccination. Subsequently visiting nurses had been able to keep up with immunizations to a degree.

Kitty also instructed expectant mothers on how to care for themselves during pregnancy, and their babies afterward. Most of these women would never see a doctor, and many babies would be delivered by an Indian midwife at home. Before the adults left, I drew blood to check for venereal disease.

The audiometer to test hearing also made its debut. Because of the noise of the ship's motor, and clinic schedules, a crew member had to carry it ashore. Lugging its 40 pounds over slippery seaweed on rocky beaches was an acrobatic feat. Kitty told us of one deaf old man whose face had lighted up when he heard sounds through the audiometer. Wistfully he remarked, "I'd sure like to have a gadget like that so I could hear!"

Solutions did exist for some of the problems, and yet we could do nothing about them. We found this a discouraging part of gathering statistics. It was hard to explain to people in outlying villages that a solution to their problem was only feasible if we could demonstrate that enough cases were present to make it financially worthwhile to treat them. Eventually the Territory would have a program for the hard-of-hearing, but in 1946 the closest hearing-aid companies and their salesmen were 1000 miles away in Washington state. Too few physicians in Alaska had the time or experience to treat hearing defects.

On the whole, the Indians struck me as delightful people. Sometimes language was a problem, because some of the older people spoke no English. I found X-raying much easier and more fun after I learned a few words of Tlingit, such as "Take a deep breath and hold it," and "Thank you." The elders beamed with pleasure and shook my hand or patted my shoulder and started long conversations. It was difficult to let them know that they had just heard the extent of my entire Tlingit vocabulary.

Kitty had problems in gender when one of the mothers would say, "See Mary over there, he going to have a baby soon." Or, "Johnny, she got sore ear." For some reason, 'he,' 'she,' 'him,' and 'her' were reversed in this area. Rex, a big tease, captivated the children on the dock, by saying "Hi, boys" to the girls and vice-versa. This threw them into fits of laughter. They knew they were girls or boys, but just not whether they were 'he's' or 'she's'.

It was hard to believe that only 83 years earlier, a white man in this area could not safely leave his trading post or fort without firearms. The Indians traded peacefully in the Russian settlements, but took any opportunity that arose to kill any white man found alone and away from town. This change had taken place in the lifetime of a few of the oldest Tlingits we X-rayed.

After three days' work in Angoon, Dr. Leo Gehrig, a TB consultant from the United States Public Health Service in Washington, D.C., joined us and persuaded Dr. Block to X-ray the cannery workers. While the doctors and I worked on the cannery population, Rex and Gus ferried Kitty by small boat to the village of Tenakee, six miles away. No longer did we have faith in radio messages to advise people of the *Hygiene's* arrival. Kitty was to organize the village so its residents would be ready when we arrived the next day.

Gus intensified Kitty's nervousness about her first expedition into the wilds of Alaska when he warned, "Be sure to take matches, a knife, and extra food in case we get in trouble."

Rex added, "Wear a life jacket, the tides and currents around here are tricky and who knows when the motor will fail? We may be stranded on bear-infested shores."

Kitty was not sure how much was fact and how much was intended to scare an uninitiated landlubber. After a safe arrival, Rex and Gus entertained the children of Tenakee with their tall tales, while Kitty prepared the adults for the coming program.

Later in the day, we made our way through the sunlit waters to join Kitty and the boys. On the way, Darrell spotted two humpback whales. It was thrilling to watch their giant bodies thrashing and lashing as they jumped high out of the water. I asked Darrell if they could be mating. He said "Sorry, they are just feeding and probably trying to chase each other away from a good school of herring or plankton."

Tenakee, Basket Bay, and Warm Springs Bay
Saturday, June 8, to Monday, June 10

Oldtimers both white and Native, who drank their pension money and soaked their rheumatic bones in the local hot springs, comprised the major part of Tenakee's population of 70. No social workers or relatives bothered them there. At first they said, "I don't need an X-ray, I'm healthy," but when they saw women aboard, they changed their minds. The bachelors remained in Tenakee year round, but the few families varied with the seasons. One tuberculous family was discovered on the dock five minutes before they were to leave on their seiner for the fishing grounds.

Dr. Gehrig found a suspicious area in a screening X-ray of a patient named Jane. He sent Kitty to bring her back for a full-size film for confirmation. Kitty found her, but she was very drunk. After some persuasion she promised to come down to the ship with a friend. Kitty believed people did better if they acted on their own volition, so she left Jane to come on her own. When Jane hadn't appeared after an hour, Kitty went back. Jane had continued drinking. When she heard Kitty's knock she pretended she wasn't there. Kitty kidded her through the closed door until Jane peeked through the curtains to tell Kitty she would be a good girl next year, but was too drunk this year. With more joshing, Jane came out and grabbed her husband's and Kitty's arms and the three of them weaved down the lane while Jane explained that they were celebrating his homecoming after an eight-month absence. I crossed my fingers as Jane clambered down the ladder. She made it safely. Sadly, the repeat X-ray showed a full-fledged case of TB. We referred her for hospitalization when a bed became available. In our first week of work we had identified 11 cases of tuberculosis.

We spent a glorious Sunday in Basket Bay, where I reclined on the deck in the warm sun. It was difficult to stay behind while the others explored and caught crabs, but at least I was there. Warm Springs Bay, our next stop, had only 11 residents and we finished the work quickly, going on to Tyee and Fanshaw, small settlements a few hours apart. We were able to complete our program during the day, and then Darrell made use of the long evenings to travel to the next village.

Tyee
Monday, June 10, to Wednesday, June 12

Tyee was a small cannery town on the southern tip of Admiralty Island. There, after I finished X-raying, I scrambled up a ladder onto the dock and left the ship for the first time since my surgery in Juneau. Dr. Block got upset with me as she thought I was disregarding her orders to keep my broken toe elevated whenever possible. She calmed down when I explained that an old family friend was waiting with a jitney at the top of the ladder. He took me to his office, where I sat with my foot up while we visited.

I was having a rough time. On the one hand, if I did not keep my foot elevated, the infection flared up, and my foot became an angry red, swollen and very painful. Dr. Block and Kitty warned me I could lose my toe if that continued. On the other hand, Dr. Gehrig threatened that if I could not do the work, they would have to replace me.

I knew I could handle the work as soon as my toe healed. I did not want to lose the opportunity to take part in this project that was so desperately needed and included all the elements of travel, adventure, scenery, and meeting another culture—something most people could only dream of. My emotions were leaping from the depths to the heights as my foot swelled and shrank. Penicillin was not readily available in those days, and I was taking sulfa. Dr. Gehrig, fresh from the Army, thought I was goldbricking until Dr. Block explained that I had a serious problem which had occurred because a crew member had neglected to clean up fuel spilled on the deck. Once he understood the situation, Dr. Gehrig also pitched in and helped me in the X-ray program.

It was in Tyee that Matt, a fisherman from Douglas, wanted his ears washed out—more to meet Kitty than anything else. In a matter of minutes he proposed to her, explaining he had a one-room cabin and $700 to stock flour and beans for the winter. Kitty turned him down. (Later, in Douglas, he failed to recognize the nurse who had broken his heart.)

The villages we had visited were in protected waters, so rough weather had not been bothersome, but other aspects of shipboard living required some adjustments. Kitty and I had small adjacent outside staterooms furnished with built-in bunks one over the other, a bench, a tiny washbasin, and a 3x3-foot closet. Next to the head of my bed, the electric steering mechanism crunched, screeched, and groaned every time the wheel was turned. One thin sheet of plywood separated it from my head, but after a short time I noticed its noises no more than the ticking of a clock.

Kitty's bunk was separated by a thin wall from the shower and flushing toilet. She also became accustomed to their sounds. Our outside staterooms were wonderful in good weather, but when it rained we had to had to cross a wet deck to get to the head or any other part of the ship.

One small porthole provided ventilation, far from adequate in warm weather. In order to breathe at night we left our doors ajar. At first we worried, feeling as though we were sleeping in a hotel room with the door open, but we soon learned we were as safe as though we were in our own homes. Even when other boats tied up alongside and strange fishermen walked past our cabins, there was no need to lock or even close the doors. Cameras, money, or anything else of value would not be disturbed. "This," several native-born Alaskan crew members informed us somewhat haughtily, "is Alaska."

Conversation was lively at the dinner table on the evening we returned to Juneau after this first shakedown trip. In spite of our initial difficulties, we all believed we could work out the bugs and develop an efficient program. Little did we know what lay ahead.

Juneau
Thursday, June 13, to Wednesday, June 19

Within minutes of the time we docked in Juneau, Dr. Albrecht, Miss Whitney, the nursing supervisor, and Ralph Williams, the director of laboratories, climbed down the ladder to the ship, all eager to hear how the maiden voyage had fared. We were just as eager to report.

Dr. Block assured Dr. Albrecht that the new vessel was far more efficient and seaworthy than its predecessor. I was enthusiastic about our 4x5-inch photoroentgen X-ray machine. It was valuable for taking mass X-rays because the small film exaggerated most details. Patients whose small films showed suspicious lesions were called back immediately for large 14x17-inch films that showed detail in true scale.

To solve the problem of delayed reports on the VD tests, which we were sending to the lab in Juneau, I suggested that I could perform a Mazzini screening test for syphilis on board.

Kitty pressed for more time for a generalized health service, with classes and time for the doctor and nurse to report and interpret the results of physical exams, X-rays, and laboratory tests to the patients. Sending letters to patients after we left was not appropriate for this population, as many of them read English only with difficulty. We also needed time to treat immediate medical problems. People who were suffering were not interested in being X-rayed or even coming to see us if we were not going to try to help them.

Doctors from the Army and from the United States Public Health Service came to inspect our facilities. Mr. Martinson, who had installed the X-ray machine, flew up from the States to check it out.

The interest exhibited by the many health care professionals made us more aware of the challenge of this tuberculosis survey of Alaska's population of 81,445 people, widely scattered over 586,000 square miles in small, isolated villages. In addition to the geographic problems, we would be facing cultures varying from contemporary in mainstream towns such as Juneau and Ketchikan, to those in traditional villages where modern concepts of medicine were unknown and few spoke English. In fact, their languages had no equivalent words for interpreters to use. Only the fear of tuberculosis was universal. We were the first of several planned units which would deliver this service by ship, truck, and plane.

After the crew made a few alterations in the clinic, our next project would be a month-long mass X-ray survey of Ketchikan's 5000 residents, a politically expedient act. We learned later that politics might not be the best criterion to use for planning a marine program in Alaska. Weather entered the picture.

Because Ketchikan had an active public health program as well as several doctors and a hospital, our laboratory, immunization, and nursing work would be minimal. Kitty told me she didn't like the idea that a public health nurse should be doing the support work for an X-ray program, she preferred educating people in public health matters, but she guessed she could put up with it for a month. On the other hand, I was relieved to be able to give the X-ray machine a good workout. Mr. Martinson planned to be in Ketchikan to check it over once more before it went forth into the wilderness. Gus and I had one more chance to pick his brains on any problems that might come up. Unfortunately, none of us projected the scenarios that brought future difficulties.

Dr. Block waved good-bye from the dock as we pulled away, headed for Ketchikan. We were sad to see this gentle and effective doctor leave. She was resuming her duties as Director of Maternal and Child Health Care in Juneau. Dr. Gehrig remained to orient the new physician, Dr. Georgia Krusich. Pert, middle-aged, and proud of her petite figure, she came from California, an unknown personality.

Ketchikan
Friday, June 21, to Saturday, July 20

We traveled south to Revillagigedo Island, where on June 21 we tied up at one of the large docks near the center of Ketchikan. Seven canneries, a cold storage plant, and a sawmill shared the waterfront with steamship docks, seaplane bases, and city floats. Deer Mountain with its ski slope towered over this small town.

Visitors started to arrive shortly after we were secured to the dock. When the tide was high, they stepped aboard easily, but when the tide went out, a major problem arose; the only way on and off the ship was to climb a 20-foot ladder. In the Native villages people did this as a matter of course. We who worked on the ship wore jeans and sneakers, and were getting used to the climb. But the ladder was a frightening barrier for many of the Ketchikan women, particularly those in high heels and skirts, or those carrying babies.

Quickly the Ketchikan Health Department arranged a space for the *Hygiene* at the small-boat harbor. She was tied to one of the floats connected to the shore by a sloping walkway on rollers. There, a giant among the smaller fishing boats, she looked like a duck surrounded by her ducklings. For those of us living aboard, the new outlook at low tide was a great improvement over the underside of the Ketchikan docks, where sewer outfalls and floating garbage comprised the view.

Lois Jund, the Department's health educator, had organized the town, making appointments for 3000 citizens to be X-rayed. Fear of the dreaded tuberculosis and interest in seeing the ship stimulated a good turnout. During the first two weeks 200 X-rays were scheduled for each day, but we generally took 250 to 300. Volunteers helped at the morning and afternoon sessions as well as three nights weekly. Five local doctors cooperated with us, and the two daily newspapers, the radio station, and nine churches wholeheartedly supported the program.

In the past, many white Alaskans had dismissed TB as a disease only of the Natives. They did not want to accept that the mortality rate in the white population of Alaska was 3 times higher than the average in the white population in the States.

As we neared the end of the survey, fewer and fewer patients came in. Nevertheless, more TB was showing up as the nurses brought in families from the Native villages and prodded those whom they knew should be checked. The X-ray machine behaved beautifully. It whirred through 3400 X-rays between June 24 and July 18, discovering more cases of TB than expected.

On the ship we had become an efficient team. It took a while to become acquainted with Dr. Krusich. At first public relations, which included speaking with politicians, radio announcers, newspaper interviewers, and other doctors, occupied her time. Then as more and more positive cases showed up, she spent a lot of time reading the X-rays and counseling the patients. Kitty had been busy taking histories on the positive cases, rounding up those whose small films were suspicious, and also overseeing the volunteers. I was slowly regaining the use of my foot, and it was a great day when I threw away my crutches. With Forrest's continued help, I was able to keep up with the work.

My first visitor was Dixie, Ketchikan's bacteriologist. Saturday afternoon she breezed aboard, longlegged, tan, pretty, and bubbling with enthusiasm.

"Do you need anything?....I haven't any X-ray equipment, but I have lots of laboratory supplies....If you ever want anything let me know....Would any of you like to go fishing on Sunday?....I caught two salmon last weekend....The fishing should still be good...or, would you rather go and climb Deer Mountain and pick berries and make pies?...but first of all, could the medical staff come for dinner tomorrow night?"

It took a few minutes to sort out this stream of delightful invitations. I immediately accepted salmon fishing because I could do that with my foot

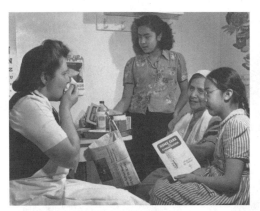

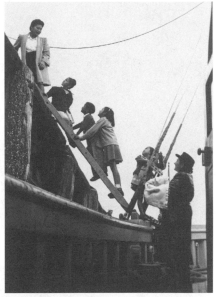

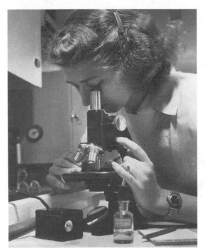

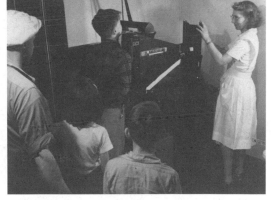

Top: left, Kitty teaching;
right, patients departing.
Middle: left, Susie;
right, Susie taking an X-ray.
Bottom: Dr. Krusich.

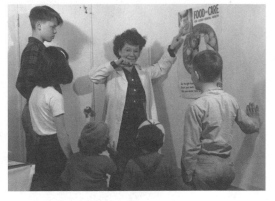

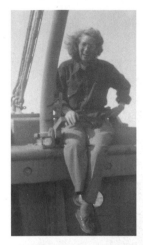
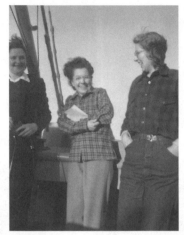
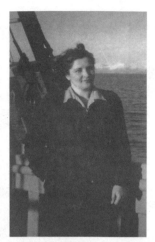

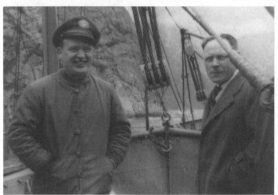

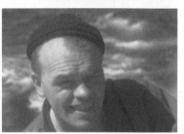

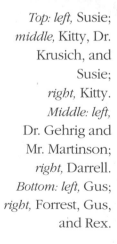

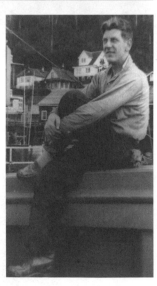

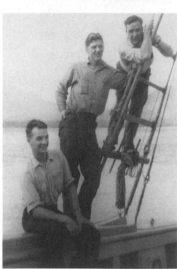

Top: left, Susie; *middle,* Kitty, Dr. Krusich, and Susie; *right,* Kitty. *Middle: left,* Dr. Gehrig and Mr. Martinson; *right,* Darrell. *Bottom: left,* Gus; *right,* Forrest, Gus, and Rex.

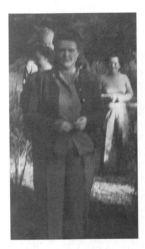
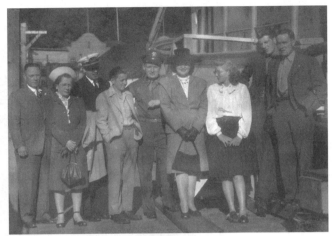

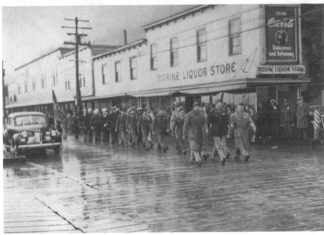

Top: left, Clarabelle; *right,* Mr. Martinson, Dr. Krusich, Capt. Darrell Naish, Tommy, Dr. Gehrig, Kitty, Susie, Gus, and Rex.
Middle and bottom, left: Ketchikan, a rainy Fourth of July parade.

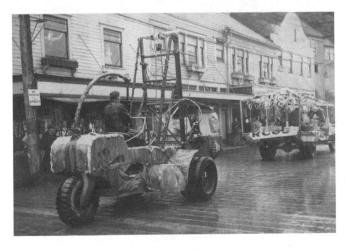

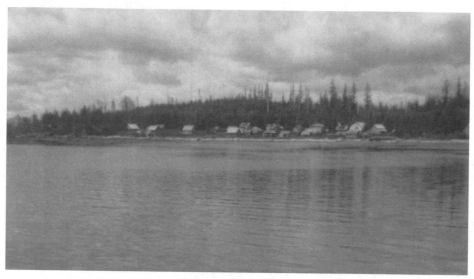

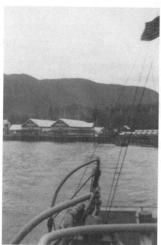

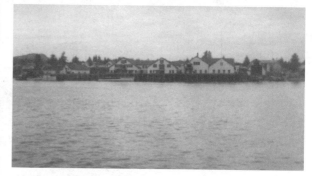

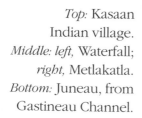

Top: Kasaan
Indian village.
Middle: left, Waterfall;
right, Metlakatla.
Bottom: Juneau, from
Gastineau Channel.

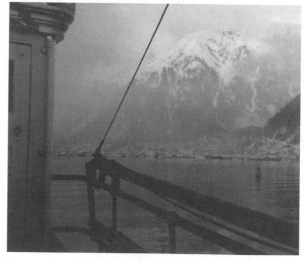

up. Our expedition ended in a lovely log cabin near the end of the road where we baked fish and pies and spent happy hours talking with Dixie and her friends around a big open fireplace. The conversations ranged from whether Ketchikan's water should be chlorinated, a hot issue, to the merits and disadvantages of statehood.

The local nurses showered Kitty with invitations. It looked as though the next month would be very busy socially if we had time free from work. One memorable night a couple of our new friends invited Kitty and me on a hayride in a truck to a barn dance of schottisches and polkas. It was especially enjoyable because we had always associated hayrides with farming communities, not fishing centers. Moonlight added to the atmosphere, and it was a nice contrast to the many nights spent X-raying. I had not imagined how important diverse opinions and activities were until I had spent all my time with the same small group of people on the ship. Even though we were still working, these social activities made me feel as though I had been on a vacation.

Kasaan
Sunday, July 21, to Tuesday, July 23

As the Ketchikan survey was drawing to a close, Dr. Gehrig and Dr. Cramer, a Ketchikan physician, chartered a plane to visit the cannery superintendents of the area and plan the Hygiene's next surveys. So Kasaan was ready when we arrived after a pleasant 30-mile run across Behm Canal to Prince of Wales Island.

Three hundred to 400 Haida Indians had originally migrated north from the Queen Charlotte Islands and established this village. In 1945 the little *Hy-Gene* had found only 50 to 60 living there. The decrease in population was attributed to local friction, intermarriage into other villages, and death. Now the 30 remaining Haidas had become a minority—the canneries had imported 90 Filipinos to run their production lines.

Mr. Peters, superintendent of the Kasaan cannery, greeted us and volunteered his resources to assist us with the program. This was typical of the welcome and help given to us at all the canneries. None refused to allow the men to come to the clinic during working hours, and many of the cannery clerks gave invaluable secretarial aid by addressing and filling in the blanks on the X-ray cards.

One of the Filipinos, a medical student working his way through college, interpreted in his own language to the other men the purpose and results of the survey. The workers gave an outstanding impression of cheerfulness and cleanliness. At night the sound of their guitars and sentimental songs carried across the moonlit waters.

A typical emergency occurred during the survey. One of the Native women slipped on a log and broke her ankle. Dr. Krusich called an emergency plane and shipped her off to the nearby Ketchikan hospital. A wheelbarrow was used to transport the patient from her home to the plane.

Remains of the old Kasaan village lay beyond the cannery and the locked and desolate schoolhouse. Miss Stauffer, a Presbyterian medical missionary who had served in China and was now stationed in Kasaan, explained that the Bureau of Indian Affairs had arranged to send the few school-age children to boarding schools.

Several delightful woodland trails led out from the village to the Natives' community house, cemetery, and a totem park that had been restored by the Civilian Conservation Corps (CCC). One evening as dusk approached, Gus and Kitty wandered down an arch of shadowy trees and bushes. Suddenly, there ahead of them sat a huge bear. They raced back to the ship in a dead heat. The next day in broad daylight they approached the same spot to measure the footprints, but found none. Reluctantly they admitted their imaginations had magnified a dead tree stump. It was a while before Rex let Gus forget the incident.

Metlakatla
Wednesday, July 24, to Friday, July 26

Our next stop was Metlakatla, Father Duncan's famed cooperative town and cannery, on Annette Island. The history of this fascinating place intrigued us. We heard several versions of his story; the one by Clark in his *History of Alaska* went as follows. In 1857 a Church Missionary Society in London sent Mr. Duncan, a red-headed student at Highbury College, to Fort Simpson, a Hudson Bay's trading post. There the young missionary learned the Tsimshian language, and after a year persuaded the Natives to build a schoolhouse, where he taught 100 children and 50 adults.

Fort Simpson, however, with its liquor and general immorality, was a poor place for missionary efforts, so Duncan led his congregation to the site of an old Tsimshian village named Metla-Katla. The area had sheltered beaches and flat land suitable for cultivation. To move with "Father" Duncan, the Indians had to pledge to forego all heathen rites and put themselves under Duncan's command.

Each man had to build his own European-style house with lumber brought in from outside, and to wear European-style clothing. The town was spotless. A special guest building was set up so visitors would not soil the colonists' homes. Policemen maintained order. The adults volunteered to work on community projects such as building streets or schools. To cover costs, a tax that could be paid in money, blankets, or other goods was levied.

Duncan's leadership was so successful that Metlakatla became a model village. He taught handicrafts and acted as doctor, builder, administrator, and judge. In 1878 the villagers had their own schooner, which made regular commercial trips to Victoria. They also had a community warehouse, store, soap factory, smithy, sawmill, mission house, church with seating for 1200, woolen mill, rope factory, shoe factory, tanning establishment, and an assembly building. The population was between 800 and 1000, with 150 school children, some of whom had an unusual reddish cast to their hair. The success of Duncan's project stimulated the missionary and school movement throughout Alaska.

After Father Duncan's death, the Bureau of Indian Affairs had to maintain the school and nursing service, for without his leadership the people became demanding. At the time of our visit, they expected the nurse to make midnight calls for ailments that had originated weeks earlier. They conveniently forgot that Ketchikan and its doctors and hospitals were only eight miles away, and they depended on the nurse for everything. The Bureau of Indian Affairs could not find nurses who would stay, even though the town, unlike any other, had its own medical fund.

We found Metlakatla still exceptionally neat and attractive. Trim white fences enclosed substantial two-storied frame houses with white lace curtains in the windows. Smooth green lawns, shrubs, lilac bushes, and holly trees were plentiful. The nondenominational church welcomed the villagers, while several grocery stores and two ice cream parlors competed with the stores in Ketchikan. The cannery was spick and span. Painted white and green, it was reputed to clear $45,000 a year for its manager. The streets were narrow wooden boardwalks wide enough to accommodate one car at a time.

Most of the children had bicycles and could pedal them until their curfew at 6 p.m. The town policeman checked on this curfew as he made his rounds by bicycle. Even in 1946, the only way to settle in Metlakatla was to marry someone who lived there.

In spite of this restriction, the community was closely tied to Ketchikan, whose airfield was located on the southern end of Annette Island. The airfield was developed by the Army during World War II. Owing to the mountainous terrain of the area, it was the best location, at that time, for Ketchikan's air traffic. Small boats or seaplanes ferried passengers back and forth between the two communities, and a bus linked Metlakatla to the airfield.

Two Ketchikan public health nurses organized the town for our arrival, and we finished the X-rays quickly, allowing Dr. Krusich and Kitty to hold child health clinics that revealed many dental and nutritional needs. Despite their prosperity, the Metlakatlans had the highest incidence of TB (9.2 percent) that we had found in the mass surveys.

Ketchikan, Rose Inlet, and Waterfall
Saturday, July 27, to Friday, August 2

We took advantage of Ketchikan's proximity to do laundry and take on supplies. After the steady hours of work, the brief respite allowed us to review the problems and results of the overall program. It was increasingly clear that we must work toward a more balanced program and not just an X-ray survey for tuberculosis. Dr. Krusich and Kitty needed more time for personal conferences with the patients. We realized again and again that notifying people by letter, after we had left, that they had TB or syphilis was unsatisfactory. Many older people did not speak, read, or think fluently in English, and a letter allowed no opportunity for the patient to ask questions. As a result the patients would take little action to help themselves.

Kitty faced a constant need for simple pictorial health literature. She had nothing to offer that was applicable to the situations she was meeting, for example, pictures of food that would be available in Alaska villages for a balanced diet. A different section of her want-list included some sort of laundry facility, because when the ship remained away from the larger ports for long periods of time, the clinic was the only drying room. Invariably some VIP's or unscheduled patients appeared when lines of dripping undies and dungarees hung there to greet them.

Gale warnings were forecast for our 12-hour trip around Cape Chacon to Rose Inlet. The crew lashed all the clinic equipment in place to prevent any damage. But nothing could be done to prevent the seasickness that struck everyone but Gus and me. I happily offered to help by standing wheel-watch. This meant that I stood at the steering wheel and kept the compass needle on the heading that Darrell directed. It was a thrill to be on the bridge, feeling the bow thrust into the waves, lift, and come back down. I felt needed and in the heart of the action.

Quickly we surveyed Rose Inlet and moved to Waterfall, both canneries operating in isolated, jewel-like settings. We had just finished dinner after we tied up at Waterfall and were leaving on a fishing expedition when we heard the cry, "Doctor! Doctor!" come ringing down the dock. An Indian ran to us and jerked out the words, "One of the cannery men—drank poison— suicide—help quick—he's dying." Kitty dropped her fishing rod and ran down to call Dr. Krusich. The doctor answered, her voice muffled by the sound of the shower, "I'm washing my hair, get the stomach pump and start."

Kitty snatched the pump from the clinic, and ran after the excited Indian to a bunkhouse, where she found a man writhing in pain. We, her fishing companions, trooped along for moral support and maybe out of curiosity.

While Kitty pumped the man's stomach, we sat outside on the bunk- house steps and looked across the fleet of fishing boats anchored in the bay. It sparkled blue, contrasting with the green forested hills beyond. They stretched to the next bay, and far beyond them lay the many islands of Southeast Alaska. I thought of the life I had left in Seattle, and the fact that I didn't miss it at all, but could hardly wait for the next adventure in this beautiful and wild country. I was so grateful that my toe had finally healed and I was able to do my job and enjoy the world around me.

Soon the sounds from inside the bunkhouse grew calmer and less agonized. Dr. Krusich, her head wrapped in a bath towel, came hurrying up the board- walk. Seeing us on the bunkhouse steps, she went in to check on Kitty's progress with the patient. After a short while she came out sputtering, "Why do people do these things? Just to get attention—very convenient to put on an act like that when there is medical help around. Why didn't he do it during office hours?" And with that she went back to the ship to fix her hair.

As we continued waiting, I wondered about her impatience and lack of compassion, and a little about her stability. Several times she had given Kitty directions to set up the clinic for a certain procedure and then re- treated to her stateroom. Appearing later in a foul temper, she complained that Kitty had not followed her directions. She seemed to be the least pre- dictable member of the group.

Those thoughts left my mind when a little later Kitty, her round cheeks flushed with her exertions, came out with the news that the man could prob- ably go back to work tomorrow, and we still had time to go fishing.

Hydaburg
Saturday, August 3, to Tuesday, August 6

Next we traveled to the three largest Native villages on the west coast, as people called the seaward side of Prince of Wales Island. We stopped first at Hydaburg, another village of descendants of the Haida clan who had migrated from the Queen Charlotte Islands, as had the residents of Kasaan. Unlike Kasaan, this progressive village was outstanding for its well-nourished children and general understanding of good health habits.

After work, Kitty, Clarabelle, and I talked several crew members into using the pleasant August evenings to explore and fish. One night after dinner we followed a nearly obliterated path through dense green woods. We crawled under and over huge trees that had fallen across it, constantly looking for bear. The sun penetrated the heavy growth in long glowing shafts. Suddenly we emerged into a partial clearing where totem poles peered from all directions. These were not painted and bright but weathered silvery gray. Some had grown little patches of grassy hair or green, mossy mustaches. Others were broken, and those that had fallen to the ground had young trees and bushes sprouting out of them.

Our laughing and joking ceased—the place seemed sacred. Our voices hushed as we thought of the happy village that had once stood here. The totems, the pride of their families, now lay rotting on the ground. Even worse, many of the descendants of the families that had lived so freely and comfortably in this lovely area now were crowded into squalid houses on the outskirts of the larger towns, where they were subjected to all the white man's vices. There they were literally "low man on the totem pole."

Farther on, we found the remains of a long house on a gravel spit. The walls were falling in, but some of the carvings on the corner posts facing the beach were still visible in spite of the young trees growing in and around the disintegrating building. I wondered where these people had gone, and if they ever longed to come back to their ancestral village. Pictures flashed through my mind of long boats returning from a raid on another village, bearing slaves, or boats loaded with gifts from a potlatch at which a neighboring chief had been honored with a new totem pole. It was not at all hard to imagine stealthy footsteps in the woods, and to feel hostile eyes watching us.

On another evening, Kitty and I took the rowboat on a short exploring trip. A pod of killer whales approached us, so we quickly made for the beach. The large number of jumping and blowing orcas with their tall dorsal fins looked mighty intimidating. From shore we watched in awe while the whales fed and played in the small bay. Soon we became aware of a faint scuttly sound all over the beach—it was covered with tiny crabs running in and out under the rocks.

Remembering all the tricks and jokes Darrell, Rex, and Gus had played on us, we conceived the lovely idea of putting several crabs in each of the men's bunks. After filling a sack with the little creatures, we chortled and chuckled as we rowed back to the ship. The men were playing poker in the galley, and that gave us an opportunity to tuck a dozen or so small crabs nicely between their sheets. It seemed the poker game would never end. Finally Darrell started to leave, but stopped for a cup of coffee. Then Gus disappeared. Apparently he did not turn on his light, but just slipped in between the sheets—with the crabs—in the dark!

He issued a roar that we could hear throughout the ship. A moment later he charged into the galley in a fury. He did not suspect us, but was going to find the guilty crew member and then tear him limb from limb. Gus's violent reaction surprised Kitty and me, and fearfully we confessed before he hurt someone. That was one practical joke that did not go over too well. Gus did not speak to us for several days, and we were both depressed to think we had caused so much real anger. We better understood it when we learned that "crabs" was the street name for an infestation of a genital parasite.

Craig
Tuesday, August 6, to Saturday, August 10

Craig and Klawock were located approximately 80 miles west of Ketchikan as the crow flies. Craig's resident population of 500 was about equally divided between white and Native. These people were permanent citizens, not just putting in time, like the cannery employees. Fifteen bars and liquor stores lined the main street, overwhelming the two restaurants. The ratio seemed incongruous for a peaceful village where children played on the streets, and housewives visited over fences.

Visiting women and playing children were the weekday aspect of the town. On Fridays the children disappeared from the streets, and the women vanished. Fishing boats of all sizes crowded the docks and bay. Drunken men in big plaid shirts and hip boots rolled down to the knees soon lurched through the previously peaceful scene.

We had seen notices for a Saturday-night dance posted around the town on our first trip ashore. Kitty and I thought it sounded like fun. However, on the night of the dance when we started up the main street, we found it crowded with staggering men. Several fights were in progress, one in front of the door of the dance hall. Quickly we changed our minds and returned to the safety of the ship.

Surprisingly, the tuberculosis rate in Craig was higher in the white population than in the Native.

Klawock
Sunday, August 11, to Thursday, August 15

Klawock, an Indian village about the same size as Craig, lay six miles to the north. Contrasting sharply with the wild-west atmosphere of Craig, its residents had voted for a dry town—no bars or liquor were allowed. One store and two canneries were the only commercial enterprises. During our short stay it was apparent that this town belonged to its people. The canneries did not dominate it, nor did a wild fishing mob invade Klawock every weekend.

Frank Peratovich, a local leader, had been in the Territorial Senate for several years. His constituents were busy forming a co-op to buy one of the canneries. Mr. and Mrs. Stenson, the local teachers, were summering in the village. Proudly Mrs. Stenson showed us the part of the school building she had converted into a day nursery to care for children while their mothers worked in the canneries. Hers was the only one we had seen along the coastline. Unfortunately, the children were suffering from scabies (a contagious skin infection) in epidemic proportions.

These people were proud of their heritage. They had moved to this site from the old town of Tuxekan and had left their totems there. An earlier Civilian Conservation Corps plan had been to restore the poles and locate them at a port where steamers carrying tourists could see them. However, the Indian families claimed their poles and asked that they be moved to their new village. This was done. Many of the totems were memorial poles—these were carved to hold the box of ashes of the deceased. Mrs. Stenson told us the Indians believed that if a man was cremated he would live in a nice warm place in the next world. If not he would always be cold.

After we completed the last physical exam and X-ray in Klawock, we headed back to Juneau, where both the crew members and our program would change. On the way we tallied the films we had taken in the last 10 weeks. The number approached 6000. Evaluation of the work showed that the tuberculosis rate of the Natives was 7.1 percent, of the whites 2.9 percent, and of the Filipinos 2.6 percent. These numbers were all higher than the average of 1.0 percent in the states.

We found that our rushed survey program was not only physically challenging, but also put us under emotional strain. To a certain degree in Southeast Alaska, and much more in the primitive areas, the Natives believed that if they could see a doctor their disease, whatever it was, could be cured. Unfortunately at that time a cure for TB did not exist (a situation similar to AIDS today). The Natives who had the disease felt doomed, but many had no concept of infection or how to treat it. The major treatment was bed rest and isolation to prevent further spread.

So the people would troop aboard, often under extremely difficult circumstances, willingly submit to X-rays and blood tests, and then expect that their troubles would be over. When the only result was a lecture on isolation techniques or diet with no dramatic changes, they felt disillusioned and wondered what good we were doing. It was particularly hard when we had to pull away leaving patients on the dock who were in serious need of medical attention. Repeatedly, Dr. Krusich stated, "Health education is needed more than medical care." Over and over she tried to impress on each person that it was not "good medicine" to wait to see a physician until the Hygiene came along, that no doctor could work a miracle on infections and pains that had existed for years.

One change none of us looked forward to was Darrell's departure. He was to remain in Juneau as port manager for the other mobile units going into service. I particularly would miss him because he welcomed me on the bridge and treated me as one of the crew, which I felt was a true compliment.

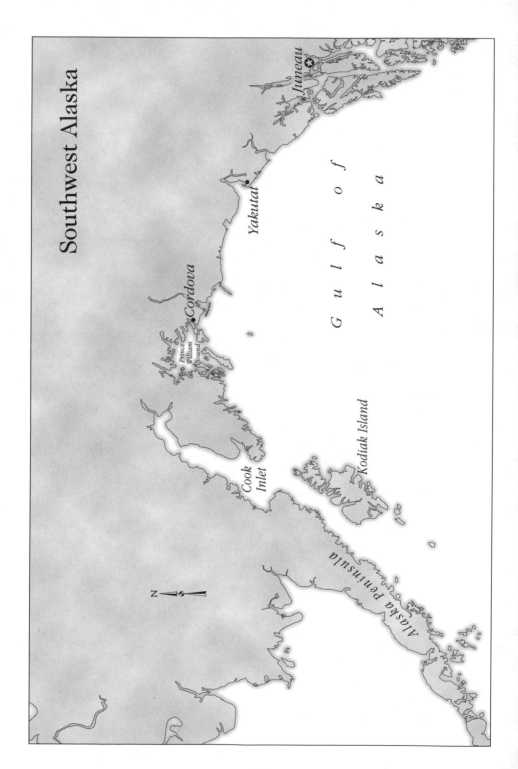

Southwest Alaska

Juneau

Yakutat

Cordova

Prince William Sound

Cook Inlet

G u l f o f

A l a s k a

Kodiak Island

Alaska Peninsula

N

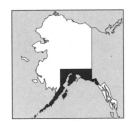

3

Southwest Alaska

The region we referred to as the Westward included Prince William Sound, Cook Inlet, Kodiak Island, and the Alaska Peninsula. To reach any of these areas by water it was necessary to cross the Gulf of Alaska, a formidable barrier to small ships, especially in the winter months.

Juneau to Kodiak
Friday, August 16, to Tuesday, September 3

IN JUNEAU WE LEARNED we had two weeks to prepare for a four-month trip to Kodiak Island and the Alaska Peninsula. I thrilled at the thought of visiting and working in these areas far from the civilization we knew. Kitty, a truly dedicated nurse, thought more about the great need for our services in these remote villages. Of the original ship's crew only Gus, Forrest, and Rex remained, in spite of the fact that they constantly predicted great difficulties with the weather at this time of year. Clarabelle decided that shipboard life in a remote area was not for her. Kitty and I had expected that Dr. Krusich would also leave, since she appeared not to have accepted the isolation of shipboard life. Whenever we stopped at a town with bars or cocktail lounges, she treated crew members to the first round of drinks. Otherwise she retreated to her stateroom and did not join in the general social activity on board, but she too wanted to see Alaska's more remote regions.

Larry Howard, the new captain, was busy replacing crew members. A thin balding man in his forties, he had gained his experience fishing along the Alaska Peninsula in his own boat. He, Gus, and Rex had known each other in the past, and they all respected each other.

A week before we left, Tracy, our cook, showed up drunk once too often and in addition cursed Captain Howard, who promptly fired him. By the time the employment office found Jessie Hurlburt to replace him, she had only a few days to inventory the food supplies and order enough staples to last for two months. She expected to replenish her larder when the ship called at Seward or Kodiak on the return trip. Eggs for the entire trip were preserved in a barrel of waterglass lashed to the deck. A large freezer held enough meat for one month. Fresh fruit and vegetables lasted only a few days. After that it was canned milk, canned vegetables, and canned fruit.

Meanwhile Dr. Krusich, Kitty, and I had to stow in the cramped clinic enough medical supplies for the entire trip. No port of call could resupply that type of equipment, and we could not count on contacting the mail boat. Kitty had to sterilize all her surgical supplies in the autoclave in Juneau, and stock a large inventory of drugs and immunization materials. I needed adequate supplies of various kinds of X-ray film, developing solutions, laboratory reagents, and sterile blood-testing equipment. One corner of the tiny lab (approximately five by eight feet) held a pressure cooker for sterilizing small items.

To my duties as bacteriologist, the Health Department added a new program of managing water sanitation. Territorial sanitary inspectors handled the work in Southeast Alaska, but no one had this responsibility where we were going. If I, with the help of the doctor and Kitty, could teach the Natives the simple practice of taking drinking water from streams above their outhouses rather than below, it would be a valuable lesson in sanitation.

The responsibility for checking and purifying the *Hygiene's* water supply was also delegated to me. The safest procedure was to add chlorine to the tanks every time the crew added water. They complained bitterly, claiming I was poisoning and spoiling the flavor of perfectly good water. I finally learned to slip in the chlorine when no one was watching. Then the crew thought I had forgotten and did not complain.

Our personal affairs had to be in order—such as enough money. A bank would be available only once or twice in those four months, even though we could spend money at nearly every port. Necessities like toothpaste, clothes, books, and craft items all had to be accumulated and stored somewhere in our cramped living quarters. Each of us on the medical staff had our own stateroom, as did the captain, mate, and chief engineer, but the crew bunked forward dormitory style in the fo'c'sle.

At last, with every cupboard bulging, every nook and cranny stuffed to overflowing, and all of this secured against the rolling and pitching of the open ocean, the *Hygiene* left port once again on Thursday, August 29, 1946.

The snow-covered St. Elias Range, capped by majestic 15,300-foot Mt. Fairweather, towered over our starboard side as we slid through the sunlit waters of the Gulf of Alaska. I was sunbathing on the forward deck—Alaskan style, sleeves rolled to the elbows and jeans to the knees. Soon Kitty decided the gentle swells were not going to make her sick, so she joined me, as did several others. Our surroundings beamed "Bon voyage." Juneau's hustle and bustle, the work of the final preparations, and the frenzy of farewell parties were behind us. This tranquil sea gave no hint of the violence and danger it would offer in December, the next time we crossed it.

The past weeks in Juneau had been so busy that we had hardly had a chance to talk to our new shipmates. Now we could get acquainted. We watched a bond develop between Jessie, our motherly cook, and Del, the new young deckhand, who had run away from a Texas ranch. Jessie's sorrow at not hearing from her son, who had run away the year before when he was just 17, eventually influenced Del to write his mother and let her know that he was doing well. All the time Jessie was aboard she hoped for a letter from her son at every mail stop.

Steve, the new assistant engineer, wasn't sure when he applied for the job whether the engines were gas or diesel, but he was a willing worker. Later we found out that he had been a carpenter. Ray, who had come aboard as bosun, had a little more experience, but he had spent much of his life on a ranch riding horses.

The morning we left, we sat around the table eating the first meal Jessie had prepared—savory stacks of blueberry hotcakes, scrambled eggs, fruit, and coffee. Jessie had met her challenge of inventorying, purchasing and stowing food for four months—we hoped.

Had we done as well? Our thoughts were of the challenges that lay ahead. I worried aloud, "I hope I haven't forgotten anything important. I'm sure I have enough X-ray film, and I have extra chemicals for developing solution and fixative. This is the first time I've ever had to think of every single thing I'd need for four months."

Kitty continued, "And we'll have to be sure we always remember to secure all the drawers containing reagents and—"

Dr. Krusich interrupted, "While you are worrying, be sure to remember first and foremost to secure and brace the X-ray machine. If anything happens to it, the whole program is ruined."

We knew that Southwest Alaska was essentially a virgin and unknown territory for public health work. The only guides available were nautical charts showing the ship's course and names of the villages. Public health nurses responsible for the area and lists of the village chiefs and teachers completed our information.

For three days we eased through the gentle swells of a calm ocean. After the first day a heavy fog rolled in, and the ship seemed to float along in a cloud, only the steady thrum of the engines tying it to the sea. I felt a sense of unreality in being a part of this small, unrelated group. We were now dependent on each other for safety, comfort, and companionship. Among other things, this would be an adventure in the exploration of personalities. We must learn each other's patterns, where we could come close and where not to trespass.

I spent many hours on the deck looking into the fog, my mind on what might lie ahead. Would the Natives in these outlying areas be afraid of the X-ray machine? Could I communicate the need for the procedure with them? How would they react when I drew blood from their veins?

I also wondered how Dr. Krusich would react to a four-month exposure to such a small group. Though an excellent doctor, she was somewhat temperamental, cynical, and sharp-tongued, with little sympathy for the Native culture, saying all they had to do was shape up. She had appeared to be happier and more sociable since we left Juneau. We wondered how long that would last.

I missed the freedom I had when Darrell was captain to spend time on the bridge, my favorite part of the ship. Larry was pleasant but, typical of many skippers, not enthusiastic about having company in the pilot house. While we traveled the ship seemed deserted. Kitty and Dr. Krusich disappeared. Even in benign weather they often did not show up for meals. On the other hand, I enjoyed moving about, feeling the motion of the ship, and looking for seabirds and whales. The porpoises were fascinating as they gracefully swooshed back and forth under the bow of the ship. They seemed to dare one another, "I can get closer than you," yet they never had an accident.

On the third day, we approached Seward, which lay 550 miles northwest of Juneau. The water flattened, and suddenly a dock materialized off the bow. The shore was still invisible beyond the dense fog. The inevitable dock lounger answered Larry's query with "Yeah, this is the Standard Oil dock. Sure, you can tie up here, I'll take your line."

The stop in Seward was to be brief. Jessie had a last chance to stock fresh food. Bill Green, the son of the managers of the Methodists' Jessie Lee

Home for orphans, came on board as our new mess boy. He was a good-natured kid who had not yet grown into his hands and feet.

The children's home was just reopening its doors. The Army had borrowed its buildings for the duration of the war, and now the establishment was reverting to civilian use. The Greens and their staff members were so friendly and kind, the home so cheerful and well equipped that it seemed all the lonely children of the world should gather there. It had room for 125. The first had just arrived, an Eskimo youngster from Nome.

The Methodists were also in charge of Home in the Woods, a tuberculosis sanitarium. The Army had given the buildings to the Alaska Department of Health. Dr. Robert Valle, an enthusiastic Argentinean with degrees from the University of Buenos Aires and Columbia and Washington medical schools, was supervising the care of 36 patients. The lack of nurses prevented others from coming. At that time, Methodists administered these facilities in Seward and on the Alaska Peninsula. (Years earlier, in a gentleman's agreement, Alaska had been divided for mission work by the various church denominations).

For three long days the fog thickened. Reports of a storm at sea kept boat traffic at a standstill. We grew impatient after the first 24 hours of exploring Seward. It was smaller but similar to southeastern towns we had just left. We were eager to get out into the Aleut villages and start to work, to discover what conditions and attitudes prevailed. Caucasians of various nationalities had inhabited the area since the Russian occupation, but no scheduled boats or cruises went there, and few Alaskans had visited the Peninsula.

Larry gave us permission to go ashore but warned that the ship would leave 20 minutes after the fog started to lift. When I was taking what I hoped was a last look around the town, the clouds began to thin. Small patches of mountain directly above the town peeked through. For the first time, I could see that Seward's flat narrow valley was sandwiched between two rugged, very scenic mountain ranges.

Hurrying down the dock, I heard the ship's engines running, and found the crew standing by. Rex greeted me with "Where have you been? We've been waiting for an hour!" Still gullible, I felt very guilty. Then Kitty reassuringly pointed out that Ray and Del were not back and that Gus had just started the engines. Shortly thereafter, Ray came strolling down the dock, but Del had not shown up by the time the engines were warm. It appeared that we were going off without him. As Rex cast off the last line and the ship started to move, Del came running, shouting, "Wait, I'm coming." He caught up with the ship and leaped across a few feet of water to land on the fantail amidst a chorus of derogatory remarks. We realized then that Larry would not stand for any fooling around.

After we left Seward and Resurrection Bay, I went out on deck to watch for whales. It was not pleasant, and even my heaviest clothes did not keep me warm. Kitty and Dr. Krusich were in their bunks. No one was around. I felt isolated and depressed as I occasionally glanced up at the pilot house and saw the crew members chatting and laughing. After a short time Rex came down and said "Hey, Susie, come on up to the bridge. I told Larry you weren't a bother, that you could stand wheel watches, and were fun to have around because you asked such dumb questions."

Despite the mixed compliment I thanked Rex for fixing it with the captain so I could spend time on the bridge again. The warm, sociable atmosphere of the pilot house was a far more comfortable place than the deck to look for sea-life and identify islands and mountains. At first I sat quietly in a corner and tried to keep out of the way, but soon I was happily steering and running errands just as though I were a crew member.

Kodiak to Squaw Harbor
Wednesday, September 4, to Sunday, September 8

Midmorning, after a night of rolling, Spruce Island appeared on our port side and offered shelter from the swells. Kitty came out on deck wrapped in a heavy jacket against the cold, damp wind. Del climbed up from the fo'c'sle, and leaned against the rail, chatting with her. Delicious odors were wafting up to the bridge from the galley. The ship came alive as Kodiak appeared in a rising fog. We finished lunch quickly, as each of us had many last-minute tasks.

Once we were tied up at the Kodiak dock, Rex and Ray filled the water tanks while Gus and Steve topped off the fuel tanks. Larry, who had spent several years fishing along the Peninsula, set out to purchase detailed charts of the local harbors. He also had to replace Forrest, the deck hand, who was needed on the new highway unit that was going to serve the villages along the Alaska Highway. He would drive the truck and run its X-ray machine. I hated to see Forrest leave. No longer did I need his help with X-raying, but we had become good friends. He was a gentle man who believed in our project.

In a conference with Marian Curtis, the local public health nurse, Kitty asked about population and incidence of disease. Marian explained, "I can't help you except to say that at this time of year the population shifts from one fish camp to another, and they can be on inland lakes or the Bering Sea side of the Peninsula. Some villages will either be deserted or have very few people there. I hope that doesn't happen in many of them. The incidence of TB and venereal diseases seems high, but I have no way of confirming it. They desperately need the program you are bringing."

On my way to check the post office and mail schedules I walked up the main street, which surprisingly was paved, a result of financial gain from the war. I checked out the two general stores which were stocked with an incredible variety of merchandise and found a warm windproof jacket that I needed. These stores were sandwiched between the many bars and clubs.

At the post office I learned the extent of the isolation we would experience for the next few months. Airmail service was not scheduled beyond Kodiak. A mail boat went out the Aleutian chain every three or four months, depending on the weather. We expected to return before the mail boat made its next trip.

We introduced Ruthie Glacer, the new secretary, who had flown out from Juneau, to shipboard life and helped her settle in her room. She was a pretty blonde and seemed a bit scatterbrained, but the men perked up when she came aboard.

Elmer, an unemployed seaman, was walking down the street when the employment office pointed him out to Larry as a likely prospect. "Shucks," Elmer shrugged away Larry's plea. "I still have $27 left, I don't need to go to work yet." But reluctantly he swung his sea bag aboard anyway. A man in his thirties, slightly balding, he had a wind-tanned face, intensely blue eyes, and a rather sweet smile. Quiet and inconspicuous, he had little to say.

Gus said disparagingly, "He's an alcoholic, but he'll probably be okay as long as we're at sea."

In surprise Kitty asked, "Have you known him before?

"No," Gus answered, "but I heard about him uptown in a bar."

Alaskan ports were worse than small country towns for gossip, and the bars were worse than 10-party phone lines, where everyone listened in and nobody heard the same story.

Again, continued fog delayed our departure for two days. We were keyed up for what lay ahead. We hesitated to leave the ship because Larry announced he would pull out when the fog lifted enough to see the channel markers, and we knew he meant it. After two days we could see across the bay; the engines revved up, and we left. Larry was glad to be on his way; Kodiak had too many saloons and available jobs that might attract his crew.

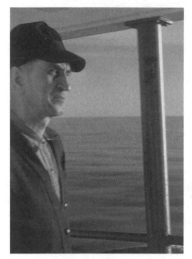

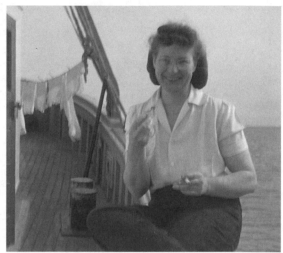

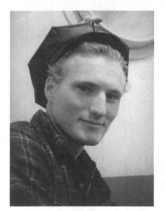

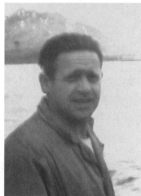

Top: left, Steve;
right, Jessie.
Middle: left, Delbert;
right, Elmer.
Bottom: left,
Ray and Elmer;
right, Ruthie.

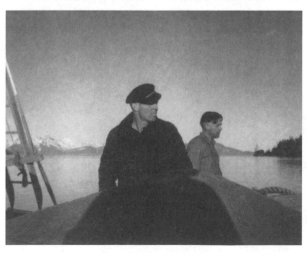

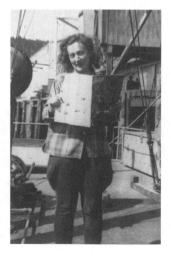

We on the medical staff, eager to discover what lay ahead, gave a cheer as we left this last center of civilization.

Squaw Harbor in the Shumagin Islands, 300 miles to the southwest, was to be our next stop. Traveling through Kupreanof and Shelikof Strait we plowed through seven-foot seas all night and into the next day. This was a dubious record for the longest stretch of rough water we had yet encountered. The ship creaked, groaned, shuddered, and thudded on each wave. The sound of rushing water was all about, especially in the outside staterooms, where beyond the doors, waves washed down the deck.

Shipmates who thought they had gained their sea legs suddenly lost them. No one appeared except those on watch. Jessie, looking pale, made a few attempts to cook. She gave up when a dozen eggs poured out of a bowl onto the deck and with each roll of the ship sloshed back and forth around her feet in a slimy mess. I did not get seasick and enjoyed the excitement of the storms during the day, but after a night of it I was full of questions.

"Larry," I asked, "how do you keep the rolls from slamming your body from one side of the bunk to the other?"

"That's easy," he said. "Just sleep in a figure-S shape with your back braced on one side of the bunk and your knees on the other."

Rex argued, "It's better to get an extra blanket and pillow and jam them around you. The pitching is the hard thing to sleep through, with that slow, longer up-and-down motion fore and aft."

I added, "My insides felt as though they were sloshing back and forth in my abdominal cavity."

"Oh, you'll get used to it in a week or so," Larry assured me.

"Or," I thought, "I'll be so tired I won't know what's happening."

For a while the seas calmed, and the fog lifted a bit. The sky was overcast and the shoreline ugly and rocky. Even the westward seas seemed different, a sullen gray. Awesome sheer brown-red mountains rose above the surf pounding away at their base.

On the bridge Larry gave Del and me a lesson in simple navigation. He explained how the courses were laid out in the Coast Pilot. Since the ship's speed, the wind, the tides, and the magnetic variation affected our heading, each parameter was carefully noted in the log. These were used to plot the compass course. The fathometer gave the water's depth, a useful check to verify the ship's position on the chart at any given time. The procedure was not complicated; rather it was a matter of the navigator being conscientious and precise about each detail.

The importance of the navigation procedures was clearly demonstrated that afternoon. It was foggy again, and Larry, who was recording weather in the log book, asked Ray to get a reading on the fathometer.

Ray called out the fathoms: "Twenty-one, 21, 20...."

Larry looked at the chart again and exclaimed, "Hell, let me check that! Yeah you're right, but something's wrong. We should have 60 or 70 fathoms. What's that compass heading again?"

He rang the engine room for slow speed. Tension mounted. The fathometer showed a steadily rising bottom, and visibility was now zero. We no longer were chatting and kidding after Larry pointed to the chart and showed us the area where the depths matched our fathometer readings. It was a graveyard of rocks.

Ray ran up to the flying bridge to check the compass there and shouted down, "It's the compass, it's way off." Larry's calculations showed that the *Hygiene* must have been angling toward a rocky, island-strewn seashore, but for how long? What had happened to the compass on the bridge? More importantly, when?

This section of the Peninsula consisted of many islands, some quite distant from the coast which itself was forbidding. Deep bays and rugged, cliffy capes extended far out among the islands. Our course as originally plotted was safely outside these hazards, but now we were in danger somewhere in the middle of them. Larry sent Del to the bow to listen for the sound of surf, Ray watched the fathometer, and I looked out the starboard window for any sign of land.

Gus came up from the engine room and poked his head through the door, wondering why Larry had rung for slow speed. For a moment he stood there, cigarette hanging unnoticed from the corner of his mouth. After rubbing his chin, he walked across the deck and dropped to his knees, not exactly in an attitude of prayer.

"Ah," he said, "that's it," and he came up with a small metal bar. "The compass compensating magnet."

Rex remembered, "Bill did a hell of a job of cleaning the bridge this morning, I bet he knocked the magnet loose with the goddam broom."

It was a nasty situation, but now Larry knew why. He had a rough base from which to work in locating the ship's position on the chart. He was deep in his calculations when Del shouted from the bow, "Cliff ahead!"

And what a cliff it was, looming through the fog! Larry took a good look and shouted, "Hallelujah! It's Castle Cape! I know where we are."

Taking the Coast Pilot, he said, "See, here's a picture of it, what luck!" Sure enough, the cliff looked like a turreted castle hiding in the fog. With this exact reference for location Larry re-plotted his course away from the rocks. He replaced the magnet over its old marks, readjusted the compass, and happily rang the engine room to proceed at full speed.

Evening approached. We were hungry; it had been a long day and a long time since we had a hot meal. Larry decided, without consulting Dr. Krusich, to pull into Mitrofania Bay—a good anchorage—for the night.

Dr. Krusich came roaring up from below when she heard the anchor dropping, "Where are we? What do you think you're doing?"

Patiently Larry explained the problems we had encountered that afternoon. He said, "I don't want to continue through these waters in the dark. They are too treacherous. We all need a good hot meal."

The nasty side of Dr. Krusich now took over. Angrily she told Larry she was the doctor, and she would make decisions about when we could change our schedule.

Larry said "I am the captain. In the interest of safety and the well-being of the crew we are going to spend the night here." Thus began a test of wills between the captain, in charge of the ship, and the doctor, in charge of the program.

Jessie cooked a wonderful hot dinner, a vast improvement over the peanut-butter sandwiches and mug-ups we had thrown together. We recounted the hair-raising adventure of the afternoon to those who had been in their bunks. Most of us were in high spirits after the good meal, and looking forward to a good night's sleep in smooth water, not having to brace ourselves against the ship's rolls.

Kitty asked, "Larry, may we take the rowboat in and explore the village? I know the chart says it is deserted, but it would be interesting to look it over."

Larry gave his approval, and a shore-party of Gus, Rex, Elmer, Kitty, Ruthie, and I collected our jackets and cameras. In no time Rex and Elmer lowered the rowboat. It took two shuttles to get us all ashore, where we climbed up the beach to the village site. We heard only bird song and the gentle wash of waves. Not even a tumbledown shack marked a former home. All the paths were overgrown with salmonberry bushes covered with ripe berries. While we gorged ourselves with the lush orange and red berries, Kitty and I speculated on what had caused the people of this village to move from such an ideal site. The silent hills stared back, keeping their secrets and giving no answer as they echoed our "halloos."

"Let's take some berries back to Jessie," called Ruthie. "Maybe she'll make a pie." We didn't have any containers, but soon we were stuffing berries into hats, sweaters, jackets, and pockets.

Having relieved the day's tensions by exploring this tranquil haven, we returned to the ship in high spirits only to find that Dr. Krusich had tried to handle her frustrations with alcohol. She had become very drunk and fought with all of us. The day had not been an auspicious beginning for the coming work. Kitty said she had suspected the doctor might have a problem, but this was the first time we had seen her totally lose control.

The next morning Larry left Mitrofania Bay at 5 a.m. and brought the ship into Squaw Harbor at 2:30 p.m., after an uneventful trip through the tricky waters. We had traveled eleven days and nights since leaving Juneau, making only three stops—at Seward, Kodiak, and Mitrofania Bay—in almost 2000 miles. The trip, while at times exciting, had seemed endless. We had had plenty of time to worry about our program. My nightmare was that the X-ray tube had suffered from all the bouncing and jolting we had taken. Would it function? And if it didn't, what would I do about it?

The red cannery buildings and friendly children of Squaw Harbor gathered on the dock were a welcome sight. They represented one goal achieved. Our program could finally begin.

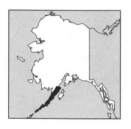

The Southwest Alaska

Squaw Harbor
Sunday, September 8

In summer Squaw Harbor was a typical cannery, employing 300 workers. It was now shut down for the winter, and only 15 people remained. Eager children sped up the windy hillside to spread word of our arrival. Within three hours we finished our program. I was relieved to know that the X-ray tube had survived the rough trip, and so far we had remembered all the essentials. I had been having nightmares that we had spent all that time and effort to get there, and the X-ray machine wouldn't work, and I couldn't fix it. I guess my nightmare was better than Kitty's, who dreamed of being shipwrecked on a rocky ledge.

In conferences with the mothers, Dr. Krusich and Kitty learned that two families had moved away because the school had closed. Seven school age youngsters remained. The parents expressed their anger and disappointment that no teacher was assigned to their town. They wanted their children to have instruction in reading, writing, and basic math, but no one in the community was qualified to give it.

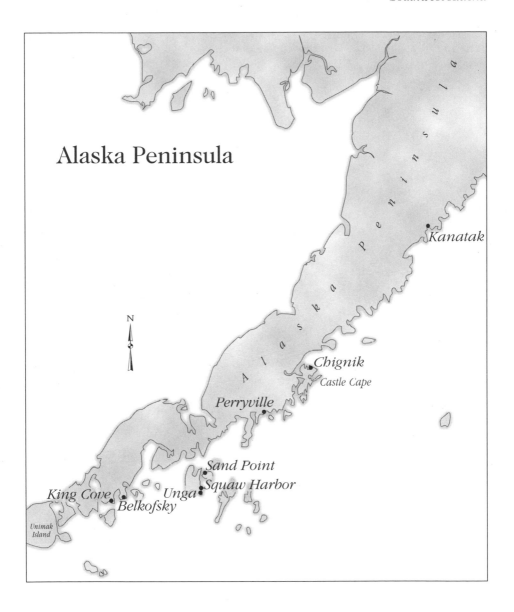

Alaska Peninsula

N

Kanatak

Chignik
Castle Cape

Perryville

Sand Point
Squaw Harbor
King Cove
Unga
Belkofsky

Unimak Island

Strong winds wracked the Alaska Peninsula and its nearby islands, whose many reefs and craggy cliffs challenged unwary ships. Cannery towns along the Peninsula had docks and protected harbors. Often some medical help was available to the Aleut population during the summer season. Native villages generally had unprotected harbors and were isolated for months at a time during the winter.

Unga
Monday, September 9, to Wednesday, September 11

Unga was only six miles as the crow flies across the mountains of Shumagin Island, but an hour's cruise by water. Larry, worried by the shallow harbor, anchored two miles from the town. Rain and wind made the prospect of the long ride in a small open boat unappealing.

Two dories came racing through the rough water to greet us. To our relief they guided Larry through the reefs so he could safely anchor the *Hygiene* within a half mile of shore. Our small rowboat was inadequate in communities without docks. Thus our program depended on villagers for transportation. We needed a seaworthy dory with a dependable inboard engine. The lack of one was a major oversight.

For many years, Unga had been the major center of the Shumagin Islands. During the Russian occupation, it was a station for harvesting sea otter pelts. Later, about 1900, the area had been mined for gold. Cod fishing was the most recent activity.

The 40 tidy homes with curtained windows gave Unga the appearance of a Cape Cod town. The village had two stores, two churches, a community hall, a liquor store, and chickens. A concrete building held the only high school west of Kodiak. A nearby playground provided recreational opportunities usually seen only in urban areas.

In Southeast Alaska, most of the Native teenagers from small villages went to Sheldon Jackson, a Presbyterian school in Sitka, or to Wrangell Institute, maintained by the Alaska Native Service for younger children. Few Aleut children in Southwest Alaska had an education beyond the sixth grade. Fishing and trapping constituted their lives.

Though isolated from the world, this small community had won national recognition for its Red Cross and war bond drives. A Women's Club kept the women busy and informed. A Girl Scout program, although adapted to local conditions, taught the girls about life in the "lower states." Two young women from the village were cadet nurses in training. The townspeople hoped at least one would come back to care for the people of her home town.

These people had had very little help from the outside world with their medical problems. In 1938 Miss Ilkins, a public health nurse, visited them for several months. In 1945 a dentist on the Coast Guard ship *Northland* extracted several teeth from people suffering from toothaches. In 1946, a group of school children sailed the 100 miles to Cold Bay on a fishing boat, where an Army dentist had a field day pulling their teeth. He left many children toothless for the rest of their lives. No attempts were made to fill cavities; it was much quicker just to pull a tooth. I was outraged at this practice. In the spring of 1946, a diphtheria epidemic struck. Three of the 17 stricken died. The Army and Navy both flew in doctors and nurses for the emergency, then left. In September 1946 we hove into sight. The more than 100 people of this Aleut village were overjoyed to see us.

Racially, this was an interesting town and typical of the area. The white inhabitants consisted of Marshall Peterson and his wife, Constance Erickson, a Methodist missionary, the Harold Frenches, schoolteachers, and Casey the storekeeper. The rest were various combinations of Aleut, Eskimo, Russian, and Scandinavian blood. Because we were studying TB and its incidence in the various racial groups found in Alaska, we recorded the racial mixtures of the people in each town. Ruthie recorded the percentage of each type of blood, when known, from the census cards (example: ¾ Aleut ¼ Eskimo) onto the X-ray cards. In Southeast Alaska Indians predominated.

The thorough blending of races over a long period of time was obvious. Some of the mixed marriages had taken place many generations ago, and in one particular family the results were most striking. The parents and most of the children looked typically Aleut except for blue eyes, but one little blue-eyed girl with Native features had beautiful pale blond hair.

The men of Unga ferried groups of 10 to 20 people from the beach to our clinics. Ruthie greeted each boatload and sent the families down to the clinic for the routine tests and exams. While they waited, we hoped the colorful posters Kitty had found and hung on the waiting room walls would attract their attention. The pictorial displays showed how TB was spread, and they demonstrated how to wash dishes and hands. Ruthie reported that the posters that pictured native plants and foods drew the most attention. All were important in backing up the oral instructions given by Dr. Krusich and Kitty, because many of the people didn't read English well enough to benefit from written instructions. The X-rays of Unga's population, surprisingly, revealed only one active, far-advanced case of tuberculosis—a young teen-age girl whose activities were indistinguishable from everyone else's. She attended school, all the dances, and other social functions.

The best course of action for her would be immediate hospitalization, which would improve her chance for recovery and prevent the spread of her disease. Unfortunately, this was not possible. The alternative was to teach her and her family home-isolation techniques, how to keep her dishes, bedding and everything she used separate from the others, and to emphasize the need for bed rest. It was important that she not mix with others, and her family and close friends needed periodic X-rays and physical exams to catch the first signs of infection. We hoped we would be able to return in a year to take follow-up X-rays.

The incidence of venereal diseases was high and most prevalent in the young matrons, rather than in the unmarried girls. Dr. Krusich set up a treatment program for gonorrhea using sulfa. She sent reports of syphilis to the doctor in Kodiak. Kitty lectured on how venereal diseases were spread.

A couple of crew members became involved in the health program. Rex was particularly good with the children, kidding them about eating candy and drinking cokes instead of "real food." They paid more attention to his jokes about their diets than they did to lectures from the medical staff or their parents. Elmer demonstrated a talent for making cartoons relating to the local conditions. These amused the people and drew their attention. We needed more of this kind of material.

Ten minutes after Dr. Krusich arrived on shore in Unga, she met the town's neediest patient. Thirteen years previously he had been hospitalized for draining sinuses in his hips. At first the condition was diagnosed as tuberculosis, but after reviewing his history, Dr. Krusich thought he had been suffering all the time from osteomyelitis. (TB of the bone and osteomyelitis are infections causing erosion of the bone. A channel, or sinus, forms through the tissues from the infected bone to the skin surface to allow the pus to drain.)

Dr. Krusich asked Kitty to give the patient a shot of penicillin every three hours for three days and nights. (Penicillin, a new drug, was not commonly used. Each injection lasted only three hours, and penicillin pills did not exist then.) After three days and nights on this schedule, plus working all day, Kitty was exhausted. She walked around in a daze, but she said she was elated at being able to do the work for which she had been trained. The local Methodist missionary was kind enough to provide Kitty with a full-sized bed and a chance to take luxurious baths in a real bathtub while she cared for the long-suffering man.

The penicillin treatment gave the patient some improvement from the pain, but it could not restore the extensive bone damage. Dr. Krusich hoped she could arrange hospitalization to give him further relief.

The townspeople, quite aware of their isolation and what they needed, expressed their desire for a dentist and a public health nurse who could act as a midwife. Only two or three ships normally stopped at Unga through the winter, and plane travel was uncertain. The nearest doctor was in Kodiak or Seward. This distance meant if a mother were to receive any prenatal care or help with a birth, she might possibly find a way to a doctor, but at great expense. Then most likely she would not be able to return home for three or four months.

We had arrived at Unga on Sunday afternoon, and the minister invited all of us to Sunday evening church services. Almost everyone went, including Rex and Gus, who said, "It isn't every day you get to listen to a lady preacher." Rex added with a wicked grin, "Especially a good looking one."

Monday evening we went in to show our health films and to see the town. As we walked down the street, housewives along the way invited us in for coffee and dessert. They were eager to hear about the outside world and to tell us about theirs. The village planned a dance in our honor for the following night. We were a bit mystified when they directed us to a large old codfish processing tank. A lively fiddle and guitar provided the music and the bottom of the codfish tank made an excellent dance floor. Even Dr. Krusich joined in the fun and proved to be an excellent dancer. All ages, from children to grandparents, took part in the jitterbugging along with waltzes and schottisches. I went along to watch but was pleasantly surprised when I was asked to dance every dance. This was most unusual for me. People did not usually ask me to dance because of my limp. Here, they accepted me the way I was. What a wonderful feeling!

The next day as we prepared to leave, the thoughtful housewives of Unga sent out sacks of homemade candy, smoked fish, and fresh vegetables. Naturally warm and gregarious, the wives and mothers in this town were particularly happy to meet with new and different women who were interested in their situation and wanted to help them improve local conditions.

Sand Point and King Cove
Wednesday, September 11, to Wednesday, September 18

Sand Point and King Cove were typical cannery towns, and they lacked the community spirit we had experienced at Unga. The 200 to 300 cannery workers who bolstered the population every spring and summer supported stores, an ice cream parlor, and even the Frog Pond Theater in King Cove. Ray was pleased that he could show our films there without lugging our 90-pound projector up the slippery dock.

The first night we were in town, Kitty and Gus went to explore some empty Civil Aeronautics Authority buildings on top of the hill. After a short time they hurried back, bubbling with excitement. Kitty said, "You've got to see what we found!" Even Gus, who rarely showed enthusiasm or excitement, prodded Larry to join us. Dr. Krusich, Larry, and I followed them to the top of the hill. There they had discovered a 14-bedroom, four-bathroom establishment with laundry tubs, hardwood floors, a fireplace, and its own light and water systems. The basement, really the ground floor, had a tiled room for clinical use. Mr. Mellich, the store owner, told us that during the war the Air Force had used the building for a rest and recuperation home for their men. Now the cannery used it as a hospital in the summer.

We wandered through the empty building, dreaming of a future medical center. Kitty and Dr. Krusich found ideal office spaces for themselves and approved the overall layout. I called to show them the perfect location for the X-ray machine and another for the lab. Gus looked over the electrical plant, and Larry explored outside, finding a small airfield nearby.

This would be the perfect hub for the medical network that the area needed. The airfield could make it a center for emergencies. Kitty, in her mind, already had an itinerant public health nurse stationed there. Dr. Krusich dreamed out loud, "We could have a traveling doctor who would fly in at intervals. If there were a small X-ray machine and laboratory, we could take care of this whole area far more efficiently than with the *Hygiene,* and no one would have to waste their time on a boat getting seasick."

Years later the Health Department did establish a small center in that building. The scale of operations was much less than we had dreamed. The project failed. Bad weather (which we would learn more about) and the lack of regular transportation made it difficult for the nurse stationed there to visit her villages.

Both of the cannery towns had docks which facilitated our work. Both communities had received some medical care from Army and cannery doctors, and the people were in better health than those living in the more isolated areas, and so were less interested in our program.

The X-rays in both Sand Point and King Cove showed a few healed primary cases of TB. These people were no danger to their families and would not spread the disease. But detective work was needed on the two active cases found in young children. Puzzled, Kitty and Dr. Krusich could not find a source of infection. After much searching Dr. Krusich found records showing that several adults had died recently from TB. They could have infected the youngsters.

Our visit would have been considerably more successful if the teachers with the usual census had been available to help. We realized that correlating the *Hygiene's* itinerary with probable good weather seasons and the availability of shore personnel, such as teachers and nurses, could become a practical impossibility.

One evening I asked Ray to put my bike on the dock so I could explore the excellent system of boardwalks. The bicycle attracted all the youngsters of the village; most had never seen either a bike or a car. When Ray gave the bike a turn around the dock, an immediate chorus of, "Let me try, let me try," rang out. Each child thought he could hop on and take off, even if the others could not. I held my breath as a couple of the older boys heading toward the edge of the dock almost stayed upright. They rejected Ray's proffered help. After they all had a try, and no one succeeded in balancing, I rode off. When I returned, a gang of admiring youngsters surrounded me. All had seen airplanes and some had ridden in them, but a bicycle was a true wonder.

While I was off on my bike, another ship came in to tie up at the dock. It was the only ship we had seen since we left Kodiak. Kitty was looking at it, trying to figure out why it looked so familiar.

"I know I've seen it before," she kept saying.

Larry was laughing when he explained, "Try putting a clinic in front of the pilot house." Immediately she recognized it was a sister ship to the *Hygiene* that was still in service as a freight supply ship for the Army.

That evening we toured each other's vessels and compared notes, particularly on how the boats behaved in rough water. We soon realized that if the *Hygiene's* hold were full of heavy cargo and not an airy clinic, we would have had a much more comfortable ride, especially during storms.

We left the area with a rising wind and clearing skies. For the first time, we could see the nature of the land we were passing. The most outstanding features were two volcanic cones, one beautiful in its whiteness and symmetry, while the other, having erupted recently, was black and dirty. Its puffs of smoke made me aware of the proximity of the powerful forces shaping the earth.

The appearance of the land was as dramatic as the volcanoes. Velvety meadows extended to the water's edge. Salmonberry bushes were the tallest growth. We could understand why the Aleuts from this part of Alaska, who had been evacuated to forested Southeast Alaska during World War II, were depressed and felt closed in. Every time the wind blew in Southeast Alaska (as it did frequently), they worried that those big trees and whipping branches were going to fall on them. The villages of the southwest were a sharp contrast to the towns situated in the southeastern forests, somewhat protected from nature's battering and Pacific storms.

Belkofsky
Wednesday, September 18, to Friday, September 20

Our next stop a short distance down the peninsula was Belkofsky, a picturesque fishing village on the side of a hill. Around 1820 the Russians had moved Aleuts there to hunt sea otter. At one time it had been the most affluent village of the area and the Russian Orthodox Church made it their administration center for the Aleutians and the western Alaska Peninsula. But in 1946, the culture of this community was decades behind that of its neighbor, Sand Point, with its cannery.

The priest, Father Hotoviskey, had lived there 30 years and dominated its population, just as the Russian Orthodox church dominated the town structures. Rumors said that he told his flock whom they could marry; when, in his opinion, they were ready for this important step; and even how many children they should have.

The fact that the marriages he had planned for his flock were not accepted as readily now as before the war disturbed him. He had disapproved of weddings between the local girls and the lonely boys in the services. Some 60,000 men had spent time in nearby Cold Bay during the war. However, for better or for worse, new faces and new ideas had broadened the villagers' horizons. "Now," fretted Father Hotoviskey, "all the girls are back home with their babies, and no husbands."

Father Hotoviskey and his wife invited us to their house and showed us lovely carved ivory pieces, imposing swords, and many types of Russian handwork. Obviously proud of their church, which nestled like a shining jewel against the golden hills, they took us on a tour and told us the history of its chandelier, a masterpiece of intricate carving and glass, which had come from a Greek monastery. Beautiful icons lined the walls, and gold and silver vessels graced the altar. These treasures had been imported from Russia in the 1880s.

We speculated that the altar pieces undoubtedly contributed to the spread of tuberculosis. Mrs. Hotoviskey told Kitty that it was customary for each member to kiss the Bible, the Cross, the Holy Picture—and even each other—at every service. The parishioners stood throughout the service, so there were no pews or benches. Small rugs covered the floor. A wall called the iconostasis divided the church into two parts. Women were allowed only in the nave or main section, but men were welcomed behind the wall. In New York this church would be a museum piece. In Belkofsky it was the center of life for 90 people.

Next the rotund father led us into the belfry tower. He picked Rex to sit on a small stool and showed him how to pull the ropes gently so as to make the bells ring softly. Rex followed directions until the demonstration was over. Then, when he jumped up from the stool, his feet caught in the bell ropes, causing them to peal so loudly that the villagers came running up the trails in alarm. Laughing, the priest explained to them what had happened. Throughout our visit, one little wizened man, frightened by the unusual activity, stood behind the Father praying volubly above his clasped hands.

No blaring phonographs or radios kept the faithful from their chants and festivals. No movies or stores robbed their coffers. The nearest store at King Cove was a two-hour boat trip away. Father Hotoviskey remained king of all he surveyed, gathering a large tithe that amounted to one third of his parishioners' earnings. If a man harvested three sealskins Father Hotoviskey got one.

Gusty winds blowing from all directions hit us in the unprotected anchorage in front of the village. We could not hold clinics ashore because the teachers' residence and schoolrooms were barely habitable. So, in spite of the weather the local men, under the leadership of Father Hotoviskey, cheerfully taxied patients to and from the ship. Interestingly, the men assumed the full responsibility of having their children examined. Mothers sat silently, comforting their children and listening, while the fathers asked the questions, carried the little ones, and generally managed the families.

Surprisingly, Father Hotoviskey had a modern approach to the health problems of the area and addressed them on a bolder and broader scale than we had encountered even in Juneau. He envisioned organized medical services financed by an insurance plan in which each family paid into a fund for hospitalization and medical care. He also recommended the establishment of a health center somewhere in the vicinity. We now knew just the place—Sand Point.

As the last boatload of patients left, Mt. Pavlov blew out spurts of smoke and ash. I asked one of the men if he worried about living so close to an active volcano. "No," he said, "we just call him Mount Puff-puff."

Perryville
Saturday, September 21, to Tuesday, September 24

We continued our journey eastward for 70 miles to Perryville, which came into existence after Mt. Katmai erupted in 1912. One of the 12 most violent volcanic eruptions on record had destroyed its predecessor, the town of Katmai. The original village had been an important crossroads. Situated directly across Shelikof Strait from Kodiak Island, it was the head of the trail across the Alaska Peninsula to the Bering Sea. After the eruption, the U.S. Government designated the trembling, smoking, ash-covered area a national monument and named it "The Valley of 10,000 Smokes."

Captain Perry had rescued the survivors. He loaded them and their few remaining possessions on the U.S. Revenue Cutter *Manning* and carried them out the Peninsula, looking for a new village site. After being turned away from Ivanof Bay by white trappers' tales of heavy snow and few animals, Captain Perry put them ashore with tents, lumber, and a government carpenter in a beautiful though exposed bay under 8400-foot Mt. Veniaminoff, an active volcano that had not erupted since 1839. The settlers remained and named the new village for Captain Perry. These people's nonchalance about the active volcanoes all around them never ceased to amaze me.

Fortunately for us and the village, good weather held. Emil, one of the few villagers who spoke excellent English, met us as soon as the anchor dropped, and Dr. Krusich arranged for him to provide transportation between the ship and shore. We started working immediately, owing to our exposed position. Fewer of these people spoke English. They used either the Aleut or Russian language or a combination of both. Emil was invaluable as an interpreter between Aleut and English. A Russian Orthodox Church was again the dominant building in the community.

When Dr. Krusich read the first batch of X-rays, she realized we were in a hotbed of tuberculosis. This was the first town where we had found a true epidemic. Some of these patients were very ill and needed immediate hospitalization, yet they were trying to carry on their normal lives.

Trying to teach families how to care for their sick members and how to prevent further spread put a heavy load on Dr. Krusich and Kitty. My workload also increased dramatically with the extra lab work and X-rays. I was grateful for calm seas so I could do my microscopic exams—it was almost impossible to use the microscope when the ship bounced.

In the three days allotted to this stop, we found that almost eight percent of the population were suffering from severe cases of tuberculosis. This meant six germ-spitting patients walked about, lived, and slept in a town of 76 men, women, and children. These active cases needed hospitalization and isolation immediately, but at that time 10 needy patients existed for every bed. Nor was transportation available. The mail boat made a trip every other month in the summer; there was nothing in the winter. Dr. Krusich hoped that when beds became available, she might get the Navy to transport patients from this area to Kodiak, where public transportation was available.

Even though I understood the importance of finding TB through a survey, I felt frustrated. I knew we were gaining important information, but it seemed so cruel to find these cases, tell them how sick they were, and then do nothing. Kitty said at least we should have more time to teach them home health care, because there was too much new information for them to absorb in a couple of days. In a letter to my mother, I wrote;

> We have had a busy, interesting, yet for me discouraging month. The scenery is fantastic, the weather has been fairly decent so far and technically the work has gone well. But I am having a hard time with my feelings about what we are doing. I know it has to be done, but I feel like a machine. The people flow through the clinic and my only contact is to tell them or the interpreter, if they don't speak English, "Take a deep breath and hold it." Then I punch the button and say "Okay." My only other contact is when I draw blood from their veins for a VD test and they are scared to death. The rest of the time I am either developing films, examining sputum samples under the microscope, or running a screening test for syphilis. I have almost no contact with people.
>
> We are gathering lots of information, but the discouraging part, and I am glad that I don't have to do this, is to tell these infected people, "Yes, you are very ill, but we can't do anything for you now." I have the feeling they are expecting much more than being told to rest and stay away from other people. There simply are no beds to put them in. Even if there were, say in Sitka, the recovery time runs into years. Many of the people from this area speak little if any English and live in a totally different culture. Some of the cases who should be hospitalized are youngsters who would be removed from their families for years. I guess it is important to get statistics so they can be treated in their own areas, but the time lag is hard to explain to them.

Sunday evening we had completed all we could do. Jessie, our cook, a caring woman, recognized that our medical staff were depressed and needed a change. She organized a berry-picking picnic, after Emil reassured her that bears would not be a problem. Dogs pranced around our campfire, and the village youngsters shouted in glee at our funny ways and at their own jokes. Proudly they showed us the berries hidden under the darkening mosses. Cranberries, blueberries, and tundraberries covered the ground; wineberries were the prize, but quite scarce. Sitting on firm, warm ground, surrounded by luscious berries with beautiful scenery all around, helped take my mind off the sad state of health in this village. At least the people who lived here had these pleasures.

Our crew brought steaks, potatoes, and other supplies ashore for the picnic. Gus returned to the village-owned cooperative store for "squaw candy," the favorite name given to smoked salmon. After filling our buckets and ourselves with berries, we stretched out beside a driftwood fire and watched the children slide down the sand banks while we relished the wondrous odors of the steaks as they cooked and sizzled. Jessie had indeed found at least a temporary solution to our depression.

The Aleuts kept wandering by to see what was going on. I heard one rather stout matronly type mutter to her friend, "They have a stove and tables and chairs, and they do this."

The Petmickeys, the town's teachers, strolled down and joined us around the campfire. Mr. Petmickey and his wife were young Texans who wanted to be pioneers in Alaska. He was one of the few servicemen stationed in the Aleutians who had loved the forlorn beauty of the barren hills. Zelle, his wife, who had just returned from Seward with their six-week-old baby boy, shared his enthusiasm.

In order to have a doctor for the birth of their son Hal, she had to go to Seward four months before he was to arrive, on the only available transportation. She had worked away the time at the Eklutna school there. After the delivery, she and her mother chartered a plane for $400 to fly from Seward to Sand Point. Then they spent two days rolling and pitching in a small fishing boat before they reached home.

The Petmickeys were outstanding teachers. It was easy to hear their influence when we heard the Aleut children drawl with a Texas accent, "Yess, ma'am."

Chignik
Tuesday, September 24, to Saturday, September 28

Continuing eastward for six hours we found Chignik, another cannery village huddled at the base of towering mountains. We welcomed the sight of its dock, where the men could fill the water tanks and we could work more efficiently.

A new community hall drew the crew for a night of pool. They returned to the ship with grim tales of the bootlegging that went on up and down the Peninsula. Irresponsible fishermen delivered large quantities of liquor to villages that had ruled out alcohol. The Aleuts recognized that drinking created major problems in their lives, but when alcohol was available they had no will power. Their use of liquor led to fights, drunken brawls, and many problems in a land where the only marshal was usually hundreds of miles away.

A few months earlier, a drunken resident of Chignik had almost beaten his wife to death. Up to the time of our arrival, no marshal had yet appeared to handle the case, and no medical help for the wife had been available. The responsible residents of these villages complained bitterly that they were getting inadequate police service from only one marshal, who had vast distances to cover with no regular transportation facilities.

In respect to health care, Chignik was more fortunate than some of the towns we had visited. Mrs. Kovich, the teacher, had given many immunizations. So had the first-aid man employed by the cannery. The latter's charges had been as outrageous as the size of his vaccinations: $25 and three scars each the size of a 50-cent piece.

Mrs. Kovich described her plans for introducing a hot-lunch program in the school. She was going to have the high school girls prepare and serve the food as one of their courses. They would not only learn about nutrition and cooking, but the program would also ensure all the children of one good meal a day to supplement the ever-popular diet of pop and candy bars.

At last Kitty was able to use her maternal and newborn educational materials. She had found three postpartum patients. One woman had delivered a baby boy just an hour before we arrived. Another had a nine-day-old baby, while a third mother had a month-old premature infant who still weighed only four and one-half pounds. Kitty had a grand time teaching these new mothers how to care for, feed, and protect the little ones from TB infection.

We were unable to work on a significant segment of the population in the survey of this town, as 40 of the men had left to go trapping before we arrived. On the last day at Chignik, I was in the lab staining sputum samples. The village chief, Henry Sanguinetti, who had been conferring with Dr. Krusich, poked his head in the door. He asked, "What are you doing?"

"I'm looking for the bacteria that cause TB, in this sputum sample. They are very tiny and have to be stained with a dye that makes them pink, so it's easier to see them."

"How big are they?" was his next question. I had a hard time thinking of a way to explain the concept of microns until I showed him some of the organisms under the microscope, then pulled out a hair and focused on that. The much greater size of the hair gave him an idea of how small germs were.

He then asked, "How do you kill these bugs?" I explained, "These tuberculosis bugs are much harder to kill than most germs. They are very tough and not easily killed by drying, heat, or cold. That's why it is so important to keep people with TB separated from healthy people. If a person with TB coughs up these germs and if you breathe them, then they can start to grow in your body and you will get TB." I hoped I had made the concept of infection clear to him.

It was wonderful when I was able to talk to the Natives. Much of the time I was so busy X-raying or doing their lab work that I had no real contact with the people themselves. I felt like a machine gathering statistics rather than a person who cared. I usually got ashore at least once in each village and made a quick tour. I envied Kitty as she went in and out of the houses and got to know people, at least as much as you can in three days.

Later that afternoon Ruthie called down, "Susie, there's a man on the dock who wants to see the microscope lady." I could not imagine who would be asking for me, but went up to find the same man who had visited me in the lab that morning. He said, "We want to thank you for what you are doing to help us." He handed me a puppy, a four-week-old ball of fur, which immediately snuggled into my arms.

I looked over at Larry who was standing nearby. I fully expected an immediate "*No*, dogs aren't allowed on board." Much to everyone's surprise, he said, "You can have her if you keep her in your stateroom and clean up her messes." Thus he removed any possibility of me using that as a reason for declining the gift. I had mixed feelings about this turn of events. I loved dogs, but felt that taking care of a puppy on board might turn into a real headache. On the other hand I could not think of a way to refuse the gift without hurting the chief's feelings. So the *Hygiene* gained a mascot.

Many suggestions came forth for the dog's name. Kitty opted for Genie, short for *Hygiene*, I liked the name Prudence, but Chignik shortened to Chickie seemed to fit her the best. When it came to housebreaking, the job was strictly mine. Chickie felt that I put papers down for her to play with and to chew. If she used them as intended, it was by pure chance.

We left for Kodiak on a clear, windy day. Castle Cape stood at the entrance to Chignik Bay, rising sheer from the seas, displaying its cliffs and turrets. Its jagged peaks stood out in sharp contrast to the wrinkled faces of nearby mountains. The sight of Castle Cape's distinctive form reminded me of our fright when we were lost in the fog on our way west. Now I felt like an old salt.

This section of the Peninsula was at its most beautiful in the fall. No brilliant reds or bronzed oranges of a New England autumn were visible; instead there were dramatic, bare, yellow-green mountains, showing occasional patches of white snow and pale yellow foliage. Was it an old land grown barren, or a new land in the making, hiding its treasures behind mist, surf, and storm?

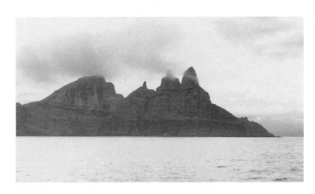

Right: Castle Cape.
Below: left, Gus, Chickie,
and Rex; *right,* Ouzinkie.

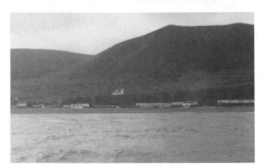

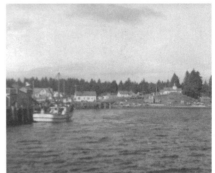

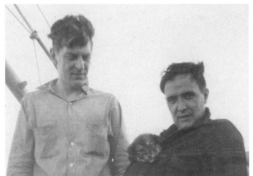

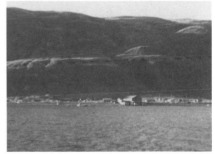

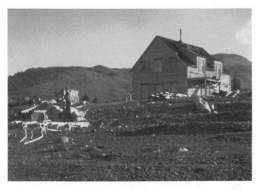

Above: left, Karluk;
right, Old Harbor.
Left: Mission at Afognak.

Chignik to Kodiak
Saturday, September 28, to Monday, September 30

Soon we were bouncing in seas kicked up by 35 mph winds. Chickie, wobbly on her oversized feet, would start off in one direction and suddenly end up going the opposite way. Sometimes she looked confused when her direction changed, but apparently she took the ship's gyrations as a part of her own instability.

The storm was exhilarating; white caps covered the water as far as we could see. The wind picked off the tops of the waves and filled the air with a driving spray. The seas broke over the ship's bow as it dived into the troughs. Water was everywhere. Strange wind-whipped cloud formations drove across the sky. As the sun set, they turned many shades of pink and then a deep red. The wind howled down out of the mountains. The stays and shrouds wailed like banshees to the steady rhythm of creaks and groans as we plunged through the cresting waves.

These conditions created hazards for those of us whose staterooms opened on the deck. If our timing was off, a six-inch stream of water poured over our feet, and we were showered with cold water. To get to our cabins from the main part of the ship, which had the heads and the galley, we had to time our departure to the rhythm of the waves. Standing in the passageway that ran across the middle of the ship, we watched until three big waves went by. Theoretically the next two waves would be smaller, but not always. Then we hurried to get outside that door, close it securely, run down the deck, open the stateroom door, slip inside and shut it before the next big wave washed over.

Larry bypassed Kanatak, the next scheduled stop, because from a mile out we could see the surf crashing on the exposed beach. It would be impossible to work there. That night when we came to Wide Bay, a protected anchorage, Larry anchored there until daybreak. The power struggle between Larry and Dr. Krusich began to steam again. She still wanted him to run at night.

The next day dawned clear and windy, but suddenly it became foggy. Ray was on watch. Worried, he lowered the bridge window to spot the beacons, but found the fog was, in fact, a dust storm hiding the lights and the mountain silhouettes. A silky gray ash, so fine it sifted through closed portholes, covered the ship. The wind blew it into our eyes and noses. It was impossible to avoid. Later in Kodiak, a Coast Guard cutter made the headlines by describing its mad dash past a volcanic eruption on the Peninsula. This was undoubtedly what we had done, although we didn't consider it a mad dash.

We pounded our way through the second day of wind and waves, with Katmai National Monument and The Valley of 10,000 Smokes on our port side. From the pilot house we could clearly see the barren gray mountains, the steaming fumaroles, and the ragged edges of the vast crater left when Katmai blew its top. This visually dramatic area was totally inaccessible to the general public. To Dr. Krusich's disgust, we persuaded Larry to spend the night at Russian Anchorage, the closest protected harbor to the park. We wanted to hike to the top of the ridge to get a closer view of this wonderland. When Larry agreed, Dr. Krusich became even angrier than on the night before.

Once ashore, we followed a game trail through the dense forest. Soon Rex saw bear tracks—large and small. That would be a mother and her cub, a dangerous combination. I decided to return to the beach and wait for the second boatload of adventurers, who were bringing a gun. The others continued on, and as their voices faded in the distance I felt nervous and lonely. Every rustle conjured up the mother bear coming to get me. I thought the second group was taking forever to load into the boat.

Suddenly excited voices and pounding footsteps became audible through the trees. The lead group came tearing down the trail to the edge of the water not stopping to look back, shouting, "Bear, bear!" I had waded out up to my knees and was looking back into the bushes, trying to decide whether to swim. The water was icy, and the shore boat finally was drawing close, so I listened to Gus who hollered, "Calm down, you've all made enough noise to scare any bear." Rex, Elmer, and Gus took the gun and tried again to reach a viewpoint, but they only found many more ridges blocking their view.

The volcanic eruption of Katmai was nothing compared to the one that finally occurred between the doctor and the captain. At the breakfast table Larry announced, "Well, tonight we should be in Kodiak, so get your laundry ready. We've been out a month."

Dr. Krusich, who was on her way out of the dining salon, swiveled around; her face flushed. She stamped her foot, and swore, "No, by God, that isn't the schedule. We've had enough of this fooling around. We *will* do Kodiak Island first. I'm in charge of this program."

Larry tried to reason with her explaining, "We're low on fuel, food, and clean linens. We won't be much use floating around out here with no fuel."

The doctor was so angry she would not listen to anything he said. So he clammed up. We continued on to Kodiak, crossing Shelikof Strait in ideal weather.

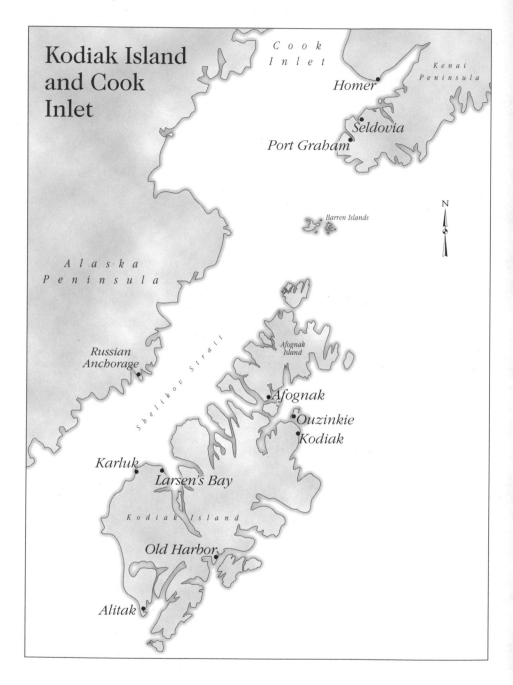

Kodiak Island and Cook Inlet

Cook Inlet

Kenai Peninsula

Homer

Seldovia

Port Graham

Barren Islands

N

Alaska Peninsula

Russian Anchorage

Afognak Island

Shelikov Strait

Afognak

Ouzinkie

Kodiak

Karluk

Larsen's Bay

Kodiak Island

Old Harbor

Alitak

Kodiak Island's towns had no connecting roads. Fog and wind often pre-vented the Aleut people in the outlying villages from obtaining needed medical help at Kodiak's small hospital.

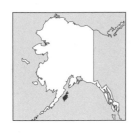

Kodiak Island

Kodiak
Monday, September 30, to Thursday, October 3

Except for Dr. Krusich, we greeted Kodiak with enthusiasm. We would remain until the ship's laundry was completed. Kitty and I headed for the post office and mail. On the way back we picked up a gallon of fresh milk, The two of us drank the whole gallon while reading the month-long collection of letters. I was relieved to learn that my mother's heart condition had remained stable, and all was well at home. It had been a constant worry, because we were frequently out of radio contact with the rest of the world.

Most of the crew members headed for the nearest bar with their pay checks. Dr. Krusich disappeared. Later we learned she had sent a telegram to Dr. Albrecht, complaining that the captain and the rest of the ship's personnel were insubordinate.

Marian Curtis, the public health nurse, arranged for the Navy to do our laundry, which would take two days. We put the layover to good use, writing reports and letters and replenishing supplies. Larry worried about losing some of his crew members to the bars or other jobs, and Doctor Krusich fussed about lost time.

Nightclubs and bars outnumbered other businesses. Heavy iron railings around the fronts of all the stores allowed drunken sailors and fishermen to roll from one bar to the next and prevented them from falling through the large glass storefront windows.

We particularly enjoyed the luxury of lengthy hot showers, dressing up to have dinner in a cozy restaurant, and then wandering around to the various bars, where we swapped stories of our adventures with some of the locals. Although the harbor was filled with small boats coming and going, any new ship mooring at the dock was a source of interest. Most of the townspeople knew we were from the *Hygiene*, and total strangers struck up conversations, inquiring about friends or asking about the conditions we found in the villages along the Peninsula.

The warmhearted hospitality of the people we met constantly amazed me. One morning I loaded a large bag of dirty clothes on my bike and started off. An older man standing on the dock noticed my awkward load and said, "Hi there. Where are you going? I'd be glad to give you a lift."

I recognized him as one of the storekeepers and explained that I was looking for a dry cleaner and laundry. He said, "I'll give you a lift to the dry cleaner, but there is no place where you can get laundry done in less than two weeks, unless you would like to use my washing machine."

"Are you sure that wouldn't be an imposition?"

"Not at all, my wife is outside (Alaskan for the States), and if you hang your things up by the stove in my living room, they'll be dry by tomorrow morning."

Gratefully I accepted his offer. He set up a rack in front of the stove, told me to make myself at home, then left. While I waited for the first load to wash, I looked around and reflected on the kindness and understanding of the residents in these outlying communities. I later learned that this friendly gentleman was Mr. Knudsen, the mayor of Kodiak.

The room was a museum. Several mounted bear heads hung on the walls, and a huge bearskin rug lay on the floor. Books about Alaska were lying on tables, and one in particular caught my eye, Hector Chevigny's *Lord of Alaska*. Glancing through it, I found vivid descriptions of the first Russian sailing ships inching their way along the uncharted Aleutian chain in the fog, or being tossed about in violent windstorms. They had neither charts nor fathometers. Tales abounded of shipwrecks, of early explorers being marooned for months, rebuilding smaller ships from what was left of the wreckage. The book included the story of the first settling of Kodiak, of "civilizing" the Aleuts, and of hunting sea otter in Native kayaks. I could almost feel myself a part of those early times. After finding a copy of the book at the bookstore, I became a split personality. If the weather was bad or the food not up to par, I would go read a few pages of my book and feel that I was in the lap of luxury.

Back on the ship, Rex was busy with his laundry project—on Chickie. When I returned I couldn't find the pup anywhere. Then Rex walked up, and there she was, buttoned inside his shirt to keep her warm, with just her head peeking out between the buttons. When he took her out, she looked like a big, fuzzy powder puff, and he looked like a proud father. She might have been a little young for bathing, but it didn't seem to hurt her, and Rex enjoyed playing mother to her. In fact she proved to be a happy diversion for most of us on board—particularly the time Jessie put down a pan of left-over steak bones. After gnawing one, the pup wandered around with it in her mouth anxiously looking for a place to bury it. Slowly the bones disappeared. I wondered where she had put them. That evening when I slid my foot into my slipper—I knew. All my shoes and boots were filled with bones!

Ouzinkie and Kodiak
Thursday, October 3, to Tuesday, October 8

On October 3, we started around Kodiak Island. Ouzinkie, our first stop, had the reputation of being the "toughest" town in that part of Alaska. Just as we were leaving Kodiak, the police commissioner and a policeman hitched a ride with us. They hoped to surprise and catch some of the local bootleggers in the act. Unfortunately they found no illegal activities, so their efforts to arrive unexpectedly failed to give them the evidence they needed.

We spent three days in the town. It consisted of 150 inhabitants, a poorly kept cannery, an electric light plant, a midwife, a Mothers' Club, a Russian Orthodox Church, and a Baptist mission.

Miss Setzekorn, or "Setzy" as everyone fondly called Kodiak Island's itinerant nurse, was to travel around the island with us. A chubby, middle-aged woman with a bad heart, she had filled in as the nurse for that area temporarily during the war and had not yet been relieved. Her true calling was housemother and nurse at the mission. She eagerly awaited someone to replace her so she wouldn't have to leave "her children."

The mission housed 10 orphans of varied ages and races.

Setzy's face lighted up as she described how they lived as a family group. She told us how the children were given household chores, and allowances, and how they learned to order their clothes from Sears, Roebuck catalogs. Later they could go to college if they showed an aptitude for studying. She was as concerned about these children as if they had been born to her. The Baptists paid for all of these benefits.

As we finished our program in Ouzinkie, we received orders from Dr. Albrecht in Juneau to return to Kodiak to pick up Miss Parker, the Alaska Native Service nursing director. This backtracking frustrated Dr. Krusich no end. Even worse, while we were picking up Miss Parker, Larry received a telegram from the Juneau office stating that Darrell Naish, our first skipper and presently Shore Manager for the *Hygiene*, would arrive the next day to investigate Dr. Krusich's charges of insubordination. So we lost another day.

Darrell questioned Gus, Kitty, and me about the problems between the captain and the doctor. He decided that instead of neglect of duty as charged by the doctor, the reverse had occurred, and that Dr. Krusich was expecting unreasonable service from the crew. He recommended that the doctor should make a greater effort to keep more regular hours. The confrontation resulted in an uneasy truce between Larry and Dr. Krusich. Darrell pointed out to the doctor that she must understand that Larry was the captain, and a ship's captain was always responsible for the safety and welfare of the crew and staff.

Larsen's Bay
Tuesday, October 8, to Thursday, October 10

When we continued on after all the interruptions, 35 mph winds and breakers rolling up the unprotected beach at Afognak forced us to pass it by. So we headed for Larsen's Bay on the Shelikof Strait side of Kodiak Island. We spent the night in Uyak Bay, a protected anchorage. Directly across Shelikof Strait, the remains of Mt. Katmai and The Valley of Ten Thousand Smokes stood outlined in the sunset. Some of the smokes were clearly visible through binoculars. This was the ideal though unexciting way to view them—no bears to worry us.

Kitty and I had time that evening to take pictures. The ship was quiet in the protected bay, and we hoped we were close enough to the hills to capture their golden tones. Scattered deciduous trees stood out in clear, bright yellow above the golden glow of the bushes beneath them. A sheep ranch with many grazing sheep was a surprising sight as we entered the bay. Setzy pointed to an area where a 1000-year-old cemetery invited exploration, but our schedule and the weather ruled that out.

In the morning light Larry crossed the low-lying sand reef or bar, and we tied up at the cannery dock in Larsen's Bay. The clinic activities went smoothly until that night, when the tide went out. There we sat, high and dry in the mud. Fortunately the ship, securely tied to a substantial dock, remained level. The only problem was that the generators had to be cut off, leaving us without electricity. Before long the tide came back in, and everything returned to normal in a couple of hours. We X-rayed and examined the 40 inhabitants in one day.

Karluk
Thursday, October 10, to Tuesday, October 15

At sunrise I heard the engines throb as we started the three-hour trip to Karluk. Located a short distance upstream from the mouth of the Karluk River, the town offered a sheltered anchorage for the Aleuts' small fishing boats, although wind and tidal conditions limited their access to Shelikof Strait. Unfortunately the stream was not large enough for the *Hygiene* to enter under any conditions, so we anchored in the open roadstead.

The afternoon we arrived, the seas were so rough that Larry turned back to spend the night at the Uyak Bay anchorage, hoping the wind would die down. Dr. Krusich, though somewhat chastened by Darrell's verdict, was nonetheless unhappy with this arrangement. She pointed out with some merit, "The wind has been blowing steadily; we might spend weeks waiting for it to slacken."

Early the next morning we again left the calm of Uyak Bay and headed into a wind that howled with increased fury. We anchored at Karluk in 35-40 mph winds with gusts of 50-60 mph. At water level the air was a wall of horizontally driven drops of spray. The deck of the *Hygiene*, which rolled unmercifully, was high enough above the waves to be fairly dry, especially on the lee side. Everyone but Dr. Krusich, who couldn't accept the sea's realities, understood why no boats came out from the town. Fuming, she said to no one in particular, "If we can be here, the least they can do is come out to meet us."

The wind dropped a little in the afternoon, but still no boats came from the shore. Dr. Krusich stomped up from her stateroom. Bundled in a big fur coat, medical bag in hand, like a little banty rooster she goaded, "Now which one of you big brave men is going to take me in?" The only sound was the wind howling through the rigging and the ship groaning and creaking as it rolled. Furious, she turned to Larry and insisted, "Someone has to take me in."

Larry shrugged his shoulders and said, "Rex, Elmer, lower the boat. I'll take her in, but she isn't going to like it."

"I'm no coward," she shot back at him, and I agreed, as she dropped through the spray into the pitching 12-foot skiff. Straining every muscle, Larry pulled for shore. Up, then down, they disappeared through the waters. We could see them on the crest of each wave; then they disappeared in the trough. When they approached shore, the Aleuts came out in a more reliable boat and towed them into the river.

Gus let out a sigh of relief, saying, "Larry shouldn't have done that. It was a damn fool thing to let her talk him into it. There's no way we could have helped them if the boat had swamped. We need a shore boat, that thing is a menace." I wondered who would run the ship if anything happened to Larry and the doctor.

Several hours later, a local fisherman returned them to the ship. Larry told some of us how Dr. Krusich, still soaking wet, furiously scolded the village elders because they had not come out right away for their X-rays. The Binghams, the teachers, helped the men explain to this angry and determined woman that they knew when it was safe and even possible to take their boats out of the river. Not only was the wind a determining factor, but also the tide. Their small boats entered the river through a rapids only when the tide was the right height.

Larry again suggested that we spend the night in a protected anchorage. Jessie, whose galley was a shambles from the constant rolling, agreed with him. Just eating was a challenge. We ate at the railed galley table six at a time. It was covered with a wet tablecloth, which was supposed to keep dishes and cups from sliding about. Cups could only be half filled. Tall containers such as ketchup had a tendency to jump off the table.

Jessie had to steady herself with one hand while trying to cook in pans that slid back and forth between the rails on the stove. Nothing holding liquid could be more than half full. At least the sea helped her with the stirring.

This time Gus backed up Dr. Krusich, saying, "We'll never get out of here if we keep wasting three hours running for shelter and three hours coming back. We aren't in danger, just uncomfortable, and the weather isn't going to improve." Finally Larry agreed to stay. Then a new storm rolled down Shelikof Strait, and the ship rolled 42 degrees. Few of us slept that night. Dawn came bright and clear, with no let-up in the wind. Up until this point I had enjoyed the drama of the storms, but I was rapidly getting my fill.

That afternoon conditions improved, and a fishing boat came out to take us ashore. Even the fishing boat bounded around in the large waves. I became nervous when its steering chain slipped off the sprocket, and before the men fixed it, the engine stopped. The wind was blowing us ashore at a great rate. It was scary to be dependent on strangers when things went wrong. Just before we reached the breakers, the men put things together and brought the engine to life. With the jury-rigged repairs, they took us safely, although still shaking, through the rapids to the town.

We were relieved to step onto the protected dock where the teachers, Mr. and Mrs. Bingham, welcomed us and escorted us to the school that they had turned into a clinic, much to the delight of the children. The health offices were two small rooms next to their living quarters. The Binghams cheerfully opened their doors, and families circulated freely, dropping hats and coats on the porch and stripping the children to their underwear and diapers in the living room. They then proceeded to the crowded health offices for physical exams. I used the kitchen table as an armrest for nervous parents as I drew blood for serological tests. These were especially important on Kodiak Island because its population was supposed to have a higher than usual incidence of venereal disease. Miss Parker, the Alaska Native Service nursing director, and Setzy made home calls.

Everyone who could went ashore to find relief from the constant rolling. Some of our crew gossiped with the fishermen. One old fellow of 72 told Gus he had never been away from Karluk, nor did he even wish to travel.

By the time we had done everything possible ashore, the weather decided to cooperate. The Binghams helped organize boat transportation and ferried all 150 residents to the *Hygiene* in the late afternoon and evening to get their X-rays before the next blow. The question of who would pay for the taxi service arose. Again Dr. Krusich said if the Health Department could get the *Hygiene* within a mile of the villagers, it was up to them to do the last mile. No further questions about paid taxi service were asked.

As well as lacking a decent shore boat, the *Hygiene* had grossly inadequate water tanks. We had no problems when we could tie up at a dock every few days and fill the tanks, but docks were few and far between in this part of Alaska. We were rationed to two small basins of water per person per day, plus that which was used for cooking and drinking. This did not allow for showers or laundry.

When the Binghams learned of our water shortage, they opened their bathroom to the medical staff and to Jessie. We reveled in plenty of hot water for showers and shampoos. At least now we had a better understanding of the Natives' problems in keeping clean. Most of the families in the villages didn't have running water, but packed it by buckets from the rivers or lakes.

One afternoon, while we were waiting for the tide, the Binghams showed us the school's museum. The children had remodeled, painted, and fenced an empty one-room cabin. There they displayed treasures such as war masks, bone weapons, and stone dishes and lamps that had been buried or hidden from modern eyes. This was the single effort we had seen or were to see of any attempt to revive, encourage, and preserve Aleut handicrafts. The Aleuts seemed farther from their forebears than any other Native group. The children had exchanged some of their collection from the sea and shore with a school in Alabama that had sent them a miniature cotton field.

As we neared the end of our stay, our routines disappeared. We did what we could, when we could, and where we could. Regular hours were a joke. We were all exhausted and cranky from the constant rolling. Local boatmen had warned Larry and Dr. Krusich that it was mid-October, and we should, as they put it, "Get the hell out of there before the bad weather hits." If this was good weather, I surely wasn't interested in the bad.

Now the comments we heard while we were doing the Ketchikan survey in July made sense. We could have worked there during the winter months, but politics reigned over practicality. Dr. Albrecht was going to need votes in the next legislative session for more money to run the units and expand the program.

Ketchikan had a greater population than the whole westward area. Therefore we wasted good summer weather to get greater numbers of statistics and publicity. From the administration's viewpoint this was necessary, but the consequence was that we had to struggle with storms around Kodiak Island and bypass villages that desperately needed our services.

While we secured the clinic and lab for travel, Kitty and I discussed the feud between the doctor and the captain. She thought the doctor's belligerence really covered her fear. Kitty confided that she herself had been very frightened on several of the boat trips to shore. We also knew we were all touchy from the constant rolling day and night and the resultant lack of sleep. We agreed that we needed to steer clear of the battle between the doctor and captain and not take sides, although I must say my sympathies were with the captain.

Alitak
Tuesday, October 15, to Thursday, October 17

On the six-hour trip from Karluk to Alitak, the wind died, and a dense fog rolled in. Larry ran his course expecting to see a light that indicated the harbor entrance. On the bridge we peered into the murk, but no light became visible. Larry said, "It should be here. I'm going to wait until daylight." He rang the bells to stop the engines and told Elmer and Del to drop the anchor. At least it was calm, and we were all thankful for a peaceful night's sleep.

At daybreak Larry exclaimed, "Well I'll be—!" Egg Island, the location of the light, was just off the starboard bow, too close for comfort. The light was out—no wonder he couldn't see it. Dr. Krusich had a new target for her anger. "Imagine an important light being out; we could have run aground!"

When we tied up at the Lazy Bay cannery dock, she marched up to the superintendent and told him to make sure the light was fixed immediately. While Rex and Elmer filled our nearly empty water tanks, Larry made radio contact with the village leader in Alitak, who told him we could anchor in a protected bay—a 20-minute trip from the village. They would ferry us back and forth in their seaworthy power dories. The relief from the constant rolling was heavenly. I never imagined the joy I could feel from just moving about and resting without constantly holding on to something and bracing.

We X-rayed the Alitak population that afternoon and finished the work ashore the next day in this most isolated of the Kodiak Island villages, which was noted for the residents' excessive drinking and a high incidence of venereal disease.

Tensions on board lessened after the sheltered waters gave us two nights of peaceful sleep. Jessie especially appreciated the respite. She was having more than her share of problems. In addition to the hazards of cooking while the ship was constantly rolling, she had been unable to find adequate supplies of meat during our previous stop in Kodiak due to a shipping strike affecting all Alaskan ports. She didn't have enough meat to feed us until we returned to Kodiak, and she had no hope of getting more there.

A couple of hours before we left, several men returned from an all-night hunting trip with a number of reindeer. Gratefully Jessie accepted their offer of two carcasses of fresh meat. Another crisis was averted. We welcomed the bountiful supply of juicy, fine-grained meat with its new flavor, and though Rex claimed it would give us diarrhea, it didn't.

Old Harbor
Friday, October 18, to Tuesday, October 22

Alitak was a considerable distance from Old Harbor by water, but the overland route was short, and the people of the two villages were closely related. The sturdily built and neatly kept cabins of Old Harbor belied the state of health of its residents. Of the 117 survey X-rays I took, 54 showed signs of TB. These people had to return to the ship for large X-rays.

Kitty found here, as in other Aleut communities, homes consisting of mainly one-room cabins that shone with scrubbing and were furnished with wooden beds, straight chairs, and bare tables. Curtains were at the windows, and icons and pictures decorated the walls. A few had rugs on the floors. Stoves burning driftwood provided heat. Babies slept in hammocks above their parents' beds. That was not a bad idea if they had inserted a flat board in the hammock to prevent curving the babies' spines. These small cabins housed from three to 12 persons, and every square inch counted.

Again Kitty faced a major challenge trying to demonstrate techniques for care and isolation of these patients that could be used in the crowded dwellings. Surprisingly, the language barrier was greater in this village than in some of the more isolated communities.

Spurred by the need for teaching materials suitable for the Native cultures, Kitty developed a miniature maternity exhibit. With glue, modeling clay, and toys, she constructed a one-room cabin ready for a home delivery. She found visual education was by far the most effective method of teaching because of the language problem and the fact that most people pretended to understand even when they did not.

Dr. Krusich found, in addition to 11-year-old Elizabeth with her obvious hunched back, two undiagnosed cases of spinal tuberculosis. She observed that these two children were unable to touch their hands to the floor, their only symptom. The X-rays confirmed her diagnosis. Nothing could be done for Elizabeth, but we hoped our visit, and subsequent hospitalization would come in time to prevent the undiagnosed cases from developing further. At least transportation to a hospital was available from here.

One day Kitty returned to the ship from a home visit to a little boy whose X-ray showed that he had tuberculosis. He lived in a two-room home with 11 relatives. The grandmother and grandfather were too old to come to the ship, but gave every evidence of TB, hacking and coughing day and night. "Small wonder that the boy's resistance could not withstand the exposure," Kitty observed.

She was outraged because the father refused to recognize that his son was ill and needed bed rest and eventual hospitalization. The obdurate man refused, saying, "There's nothing wrong with him, he isn't sick." The boy's mother, tears gleaming in her eyes in the dim light of the kerosene lamp, begged her husband at least to admit that the boy was ill. The father staunchly maintained, "My son is not ill." The village chief, who was also the father's uncle, tried to persuade him, but he too failed. It was as though admitting the presence of TB was a death sentence.

Kitty and Dr. Krusich visited the midwife to inspect her facilities. What they found appalled them. As well as being a delivery room and maternity ward, the small hut was inhabited by an old man who was an active TB case with a positive sputum. Expectant mothers came there from all over the islands to deliver their babies. Kitty and Dr. Krusich shuddered to think of the defenseless babies born in that contaminated shack. At the time we were there, three midwives were expecting six prenatals to deliver within two weeks.

On October 22 we headed back to Kodiak through a light snowfall that melted as it came down. We were all depressed at having to leave this concentration of disease. The sick people in this one village could have kept a nurse and doctor busy and filled many hospital beds. Yet we had to leave them after four days.

Kitty said "I'm almost afraid to come back here. The people are going to be even more depressed now they know they have TB. No wonder they have drinking problems!"

For the first time in their long and not always agreeable association, Dr. Krusich and Kitty lamented together as they sat snug and warm drinking coffee in the galley. Kitty sighed, "How will this many contagious cases ever be controlled unless they're put in a sanitarium?"

Dr. Krusich asked, "Did you ever hear the argument that you shouldn't hospitalize patients with far advanced TB, since it won't prevent their deaths? But we can't prevent the spread of tuberculosis if these patients are left here in these crowded homes. The Legislature and Congress simply have to appropriate money before even a dent can be made. Discouraging as it is, we have to gather the statistics. There's no doubt about it, Alaska is in the midst of a TB epidemic!"

Kodiak
Tuesday, October 22, to Saturday, October 26

When we docked at Kodiak, the shipping strike was the main topic of conversation. Sugar, cooking oil, and meat were in short supply, although reindeer were plentiful on the island. These animals were about the size of a small cow and cost about $15 apiece. Jessie had purchased several more, and the carcasses were hanging on the fantail where the cool weather kept them from spoiling. Kodiak residents and storekeepers worried about their dwindling supplies because merchandise of all kinds was disappearing, and no one knew how long the strike would last.

Shortly after we docked, a young man whom I had met the last time we were in port invited me to a formal dance at the Chief's Club. I was not at all sure a blue-jeaned, windblown tomboy could be transformed into a proper young lady, but I accepted the invitation. Then I worried. I wouldn't know anyone but my date, and I really didn't know him very well. I had a formal dress and all the trimmings tucked away in a suitcase, unused since I left Seattle, but my hair was a mess, my fingernails broken—oh dear, why had I ever said yes?

After several hours of preparation Kitty asked, "Do you have an evening wrap?" I looked at her in consternation. "Oh my gosh, I don't even have a coat, only a ski jacket."

Jessie offered her coat. I slipped my arms into the sleeves and it went on, but I was afraid to move; it was too tight. She cautioned, "Just don't put it on till you've climbed the ladder." That was a problem I had not yet considered—climbing that ladder in a long dress.

Larry checked the tide charts. I would be leaving on a high tide and would only have to negotiate a few rungs. Finally, with help and advice from Kitty, Jessie, and Ruthie, I was ready to go. As I stood on the dock, clean, perfumed, and jeweled in my pretty long dress and tight borrowed coat, I felt like Cinderella ready for the ball.

It was a grand evening. My date was attentive, the food and music were good, and it seemed as if everyone went out of their way to see that I had a good time. Part of my enthusiasm may have come from the stark contrast to my life of the last few weeks.

While I was eager to meet people and explore life away from the ship, Kitty and Gus were becoming more involved with one another.

Kitty wrote to her father.

> It's hard to tell how serious it is, but Gus thinks we should get married when we get back to Juneau. He's a peach and the real mainstay of the boat. His dry humor often averts a blow up between the staff and crew. I like him tremendously—but so far that's all. When I do something he doesn't like, like telling the captain he is handling our funds the wrong way paying our bills instead of charging them through the main office Gus storms, "You should stay in your nursing field and not mess in the clerk's job." He gets so hopping mad, he takes it out on everyone else, and then there is another argument.
>
> Life on the *Hygiene* isn't all it seems. If it weren't for Sue and the fact I believe in the Health Department and Dr. Albrecht seeing the light someday, I'd have told them to go to blazes long ago. I guess some of the trouble comes from being cooped together in such a small space. The weather doesn't help either. Oh well—

While Kitty and Gus were having serious thoughts about marriage, Ruthie was at the other end of the spectrum. She was pretty, happy-go-lucky, and very attractive to males of all ages. She had so many dates that she would ask Steve to show one out through the engine room while she greeted another in the galley.

The stop in Kodiak was to have been brief, for refueling and resupplying, and Larry was eager to leave this town with all its bars and temptations for the crew, so he moved to Ouzinkie, hoping to be close to Afognak when a break came in the weather.

Afognak
Sunday, October 27, to Monday, October 28

Although the waves slapped angrily at the ship the next morning, we left the protection of Ouzinkie's harbor for Afognak and anchored among its reefs at 8 a.m. The village stretched three miles along the beach; its front yard of rocks was a challenge for any captain. The beach was close, so Dr. Krusich talked Rex into rowing her ashore. The offshore wind was so strong that when they pulled out from the shelter of the *Hygiene*, they were stopped dead. The doctor admitted that she was scared stiff but did not want her fear to stop the program. It was true that the more frightened she was, the more stubborn she became. We admired her determination to get the job done but felt she carried it to extremes.

After several hours, two boats came out from the village. They patched our ailing three-horsepower outboard and used it on a dory furnished by the mission to transport Dr. Krusich and some of the staff to shore. By nightfall, thanks to resident Hans Olsen's ferry service, we had X-rayed the entire village of 150 people. This was quite a feat because messengers had to bicycle along the three miles of this unusually extended community to issue the call to the clinic. Usually school or church bells summoned villagers, but here the wind would have muffled the sound. The work at Afognak went smoothly and quickly because the people were relatively healthy.

Kitty had been particularly eager to reach Afognak because a missionary from her home town of Altoona was stationed there. They had not known each other very well in Pennsylvania, but now 5000 miles from home, they met as long-lost friends. Because of our busy schedule, Kitty had time for a very brief visit and then had to dash away.

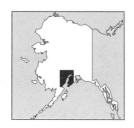

Cook Inlet

Cook Inlet presented the problem of the second greatest tidal flows in the world plus cold weather and snow after October. The inner end of the inlet usually froze sometime in November.

Seldovia and Port Graham
Tuesday, October 29, to Friday, November 8

After dropping Miss Setzekorn off in Ouzinkie, we left for Cook Inlet, the next geographical unit on the program. Most of us were ambivalent about this section of our schedule. At the northeast end of the inlet lay Anchorage—the big city, a goal we hoped to reach for the Thanksgiving holidays, before we learned the Inlet could freeze any time after November 1.

On the negative side, Larry had never been there, few of the towns on our schedule had docks, and the tides in Cook Inlet are the second highest in the world, after the Bay of Fundy. We were worn out from the irregular hours, lack of sleep, and stress of the last two months' work. What lay ahead did not sound promising.

Gus insisted, "It's crazy to go up there now. They cancel insurance on fishing boats after September. In the bar they said that only three captains were damn fools enough to try going up the Inlet this time of year. One was ours."

Larry defended himself, "Well, there's no harm in giving it a try."

Dr. Krusich ended the discussion with a definite, "We are going!"

The 150-mile trip from Ouzinkie to Seldovia started auspiciously with peaceful seas and a beautiful sunrise. While Jessie fixed lunch the wind picked up. In no time, the waves became very high, and our course had us taking them broadside. Suddenly the ship took a severe roll, and everything in the galley went tumbling—even the flour bin flew across the deck. Jessie called for help as she struggled to contain her equipment. Steve secured the flour bin. Then the ship took an even greater roll, and the galley range broke loose from its hold-down bolts.

Steve called Gus to turn off the oil. Then he rushed topside and secured a four-by-four he had stowed away. He and Gus wedged it between the bulkhead and the stove, thus preventing any further movement. The engineers saved the day that time. Jessie, having become an excellent sailor, kept her head throughout the whole incident. Several others, however, were sure the ship was going to roll over.

Following this violent introduction to Cook Inlet, we made our way into the relative quiet of Seldovia's harbor. Even in the harbor, peace eluded the tired crew. The town lights glowed dimly through a downpour, and the waters of the bay fumed angrily. Gratefully we hugged the dock as the lines went up and over. The weary crew discussed the damage as they sipped coffee. Then like a hollow echo, a voice floated down from the dock.

"Halloo—hello there, *Hygiene*, would you please move away from my dock? Ooh-hoo would you please...." wailed the voice. Poor Larry and the boys. Back to work. The huddle of fishing boats in the middle of the bay was understandable now. The dock was too weak and the storm too strong. Its owner, Mrs. Anderson, feared the pilings would give way.

After dinner, the rain stopped and the wind died. All of us except Dr. Krusich and those on watch loaded into our dinghy and went ashore to see Seldovia. The town had no streets or cars, just a network of boardwalks, some high above the ground, crossing ravines and gullies. The crew members headed for the bars, the only places to relax. Kitty and I visited Miss Jacobsen (Jakie), the public health nurse who would be joining us on the trip up Cook Inlet, her territory.

Jakie, a slender outspoken Norwegian, repeated how crazy it was to try to go up the Inlet this late in the year. "These are the worst waters in Alaska, and they almost always freeze over by November 6." She warned of hidden rocks and reefs, of ferocious currents and rips. They were why the Army had chosen the Alaska Railroad and airlifts to move supplies from Seward to Anchorage instead of using freighters in Cook Inlet.

Kitty and I, concerned about Jakie's messages, found the rest of the crew at Joe's Bar and Barber Shop. The bar had a counter that ended at his barber chair. Two old-fashioned dining room tables, piled high with the latest newspapers and magazines, had their place across the room. There, in comfortable chairs, those who were not soaking up liquor at the bar soaked in the news of the past three months. We had not seen a newspaper or had decent radio reception around Kodiak Island or on the Alaska Peninsula. The articles about wars, strikes, scarcities, and politics were from another world. We sat around the stove, warm and comfortable, until a local fisherman came in with news of the immediate world. The wind was picking up again.

Reluctantly we left the friendly bar and headed back to the skiff. There we found good-sized waves breaking on the beach. Gus said, "We'd better try getting out with three people first." In spite of the lightened load, Gus, Rex, and Elmer were drenched when the waves washed over the boat and swamped it. At this point, Ruthie, who had been quite apprehensive, noticed a flashlight blinking on the *Hygiene*.

"That's a message in Morse code," she said in a relieved voice. "I can read it—that's an S, now a T A Y" and she proceeded to spell out "stay ashore, OK here." Then she took a flashlight and blinked back "OK."

Cold, shivering, soaked to the skin, and very grateful for Ruthie's heretofore unknown knowledge, we traipsed back and rented all of the empty hotel rooms. Before we went to them, Joe the friendly bartender gave each of us a hot buttered rum and stoked up the fire in the potbellied stove where we stood around drying our clothes and telling stories. He knew the rooms we had rented weren't much warmer than the sleet outdoors.

The next day we heard what happened while we were asleep. Gus woke up about 1 a.m. and heard no wind. He worried about the skipper out on the *Hygiene*, more or less alone, so he pulled Elmer out of bed, and with difficulty the two of them made it back to the ship.

Larry greeted them. "Who in hell was that trying to signal?" "Ruthie" was the answer. Then Larry understood. He was furious when no one showed up in response to his actual message, "Come back at once." He was in trouble because the anchor was dragging, and the ship was drifting uncomfortably close to the rocks. He did not have enough help on board to weigh anchor and move. The situation was critical when Gus and Elmer arrived. With their help, Larry moved to a safer anchorage to ride out the storm.

Ruthie had read just what she wanted to believe. Her moment of glory vanished. When she returned to the ship she was in trouble. Very angry at her deception, Larry told her the ship came close to going on the rocks because of her irresponsibility.

The following morning, Larry told Dr. Krusich that he and Gus were taking the small boat in to talk to Mrs. Anderson about tying up at the dock so that work could proceed. Dr. Krusich replied, "With your line, you'll charm her into anything."

Ashore, Larry turned on his personality, and Mrs. Anderson, a middle-aged woman, invited the two men in for coffee. After a short time Larry and Gus came back laughing, with the good news that we could tie up at the dock immediately, and Mrs. Anderson was just a poor misunderstood lady. She would help in any way she could if it was a program for the good of the town. We found her to be a topnotch volunteer during the X-raying.

While the men made docking arrangements, Kitty and I explored Seldovia. In summer it was a thriving fishing town with three canneries. Four hundred residents lived here year around. Spectacular snow-covered mountains framed the attractively painted houses. The town had no movie, no decent restaurant, and no soda fountain. But it did have a splendid hospital, a good school, a fine library, and active civic and social clubs.

Again the shipping strike was the main topic of conversation and concern. No freighters had come for two months, and several stores displayed bare shelves. They were flying in canned milk for babies, but a stretch of bad weather could stop that. The bars did not appear to have a shortage of supplies.

The temperature dropped, and it started to snow. Kitty and I, remembering how cold we had been the night before, spent most of our money on heavy wool shirts and socks. The storekeepers and people on the streets had heard the *Hygiene* was heading up the inlet. They advised us that it was the wrong thing to do and very dangerous. Kitty and I reported these warnings to the doctor and Larry when we returned to X-ray the school children that afternoon.

The doctor was adamant about going to Tyonek. That was the schedule, and neither wind nor high waves would keep her from it. Larry, sick of arguing with her, said he would continue until he felt it would be unsafe.

After some of our recent adventures, I wondered what it would take to make him feel endangered.

November 1, covered with snow, the *Hygiene* left Seldovia and headed for Tyonek across Cook Inlet and north toward Anchorage. Twenty minutes after leaving the shelter of land, we felt the full force of gale winds, strong tidal currents, and a blinding snowstorm. The ship pounded, bucked, and twisted. Waves leapt over the bow and swept over the clinic roof. The bosun was at the wheel. As each huge wave struck the bridge windows, he would duck, and the ship would go off course. The seas were 16 to 20 feet high, and owing to the extreme tides in the area, they were very steep and close together. We were taking a terrible beating. I was scared, but I was glad to be on the bridge where I knew what was happening. When I was involved, as when Larry suggested that I take the wheel part of the time, I didn't have time to be frightened.

After three hours of pounding, and with water leaking into her stateroom, Dr. Krusich sent word for Larry to come and see her, but he could not leave the pilot house. Pale and terrified, she staggered up to the bridge and begged him to turn back. It was obviously futile to continue. We would not be able to find shelter at Tyonek or any of the other villages. Work would be impossible even if we could get there.

Larry called Gus and asked him to stand by. He was going to try to turn around when he had a chance. This maneuver would be difficult. The larger waves, steep and close together, were higher than the *Hygiene*. While we headed into such seas, we had a rough time, but we were not in imminent danger. However, taking them broadside presented some risk. Fortunately, waves came in groups of two or three large ones and then a few smaller ones. Larry would attempt the turn between the sets of larger waves.

To further complicate the situation it was snowing so heavily that the waves only became visible as they reached the bow of the ship. This forced Larry to continue slowly plowing through 20-foot seas and 40-knot winds. Finally a slight lull in the snowfall enabled him to see far enough ahead to find a flatter spot for his turn. Grim-faced and jaws clenched, Larry took the wheel. When he finally swung the helm over and started the turn, the sensation was sickening. The boat changed from its violent up and down motion to a few steep rolls on the smaller waves that still towered high. Relief came when the ship went back to plunging as the waves came under and over the stern. We scooted back to safety at 16 knots, shoved along by following seas.

Soon Kitty was able to leave her stateroom, and Gus came up from the engine room, and they shared experiences. Kitty shivered as she recounted,

"The water came pouring through my closed porthole and door. That has never happened before. Even the bunk boards seemed to be moving as though they might separate. I felt trapped. I couldn't get out of my stateroom to see what was happening to the rest of the ship. How was it in the engine room?"

Gus shrugged in his usual stoic manner, "If it hadn't been Larry on the bridge, I'd have been a hell of a lot more worried. It's a good thing we're going back. And by the way, don't ever worry about me if we ever have to abandon ship. I'll get out safely. I'm not going to give up after suffering through the longest courtship any girl ever had!"

Another argument almost erupted. "What do you mean—long?" Kitty demanded. "It's only been a few months."

Gus patiently explained, "Think in terms of miles and all the ups and downs of the storms." Kitty left in haste, overcome by losing another argument and silently laughing at her stoic suitor.

When we returned to Seldovia, despite the short notice, Dr. Krusich, with Jakie's help, rounded up more Seldovians for us to X-ray while the storm blew itself out. People came, but the survey X-rays I took were very poor. Soon they were so bad that the doctor could no longer read them. The violent pounding of the waves had apparently damaged the X-ray tube, even though it had remained securely braced.

Gus and I checked everything the instruction manual and directions offered. Nothing was obviously wrong. The next step was to call Mr. Martinson, the X-ray specialist in Seattle, for help. I had had nightmares of such a situation happening from the time I started the job. This surpassed my worst fears. In this area I could not just pick up the phone and call Marty and tell him what had happened. The only way to communicate was to send a collect telegram via ship-to-shore radio, then wait three days for an answer.

When the answer came, it was obvious that Marty did not have the picture, that the tube had been working with no difficulties until after the violent shaking it had gone through. His message was brief: "Pick up new tube in Homer in four days." That was all. I was sick, and wailed, "We'll just wreck another tube. I'm sure the tube was blown by a short circuit, and it will probably do the same to the new one." No one understood my concern, not even Kitty. I felt terribly alone.

During the waiting period, we shuttled back and forth between Homer, Seldovia, and Port Graham. We did whatever parts of the medical program we could, getting a few readable large X-rays, and then none. After four long days, the new tube arrived in Homer. With it came routine installation directions. I worried, "Oh if I could only talk to Marty; these tubes are too expensive to blow out like light bulbs."

The orders were to install it. Gus shrugged his shoulders and with Larry's help started to remove the old tube. I hovered over them like a mother hen. Suddenly Gus said, "Aha, here it is, a little wire not connected to anything." They fastened the wire where it belonged, put the old machine back together, and I tried again to take pictures. This time I was able to take X-rays, but they were of very poor quality. The open circuit had damaged the tube. So the men continued removing the old tube and installed the new one, which functioned properly. I was greatly relieved that they had found the disconnected wire before it had ruined the new tube.

Naturally, the weather improved while we waited for the X-ray tube. Snow covered the ground, and all the mountains across the inlet stood out clearly. During the day they were beautifully white, but at sunrise and sunset the white changed to a vibrant pink, and for a few minutes the whole world, sky, land, and water, became rosy.

However the food situation was less than rosy. Every day the town's stores had less food. Most of the shelves remained empty, and the shipping strike was still in progress. Eggs, canned vegetables, fruits, and meats were gone. Flour was getting low, and the only staple left in any quantity was sugar. The main event of the day was the arrival of a plane from Anchorage with canned milk for babies, or a fishing boat from Homer with some fresh vegetables. Jessie had trouble putting decent meals on the table. Reindeer were not available in Seldovia. When she had only two meat dishes left, she sighed, "I wish some of those shipping company executives or strikers had my job. I wonder if they have any idea of what they are doing to us and these poor people who live here."

Larry had tracked down a quarter of beef in Homer, which gave Jessie a brief respite. I was still reading about Baranof's adventures in the 1790s and did not make myself popular when I kept telling my shipmates how much better off we were than the early Russian settlers, whose yearly ship was often lost with all supplies, and who were attacked by hostile Natives when they went hunting for meat, and how they had craved tea and tobacco and often went years without any, and.... "That's enough, Susie!" they chimed in. "We get the picture."

Homer and Port Graham
Saturday, November 9, to Friday, November 15

Homer differed from the isolated, compact coastal villages with stable or declining populations that we had been visiting. The town, soon to be connected to Seward and Anchorage by a highway, was the hub of a 500,000-acre agricultural and stock-raising district. An influx of farmers and homesteaders from the Midwest had rapidly increased the population. The newcomers had built roads that were not much more than muddy tracks, but they were able to get about in their trucks and visit each other.

A five-mile-long sandspit separated Kachemak Bay from Cook Inlet. Homer, located at the base of the spit, had no decent anchorage. A rickety dock, linked to the town by four miles of road, perched just inside the outer end of the spit. The low spit broke the force of the waves from the inlet but gave no protection from the wind. Jakie advised Larry that this was the best place for patients to reach the clinic. The wharf manager assured Larry the pier was stronger than it looked, and that he had plenty of water. Larry took his word for it and tied up to the leeward side of the dock.

We were in the clinic setting things up when all of a sudden something did not feel right. The ship's normal motion was gone, and the deck was no longer level. Gus, Rex, and Larry, who had been below helping us, dashed up and found we were hard aground. Gus started the engines immediately, but the ship did not budge. The tide still had two hours to run out.

The force of the wind on the port side had given us a decided list to starboard and away from the dock. The ship's angle became steadily and rapidly worse. The men fastened more lines to the dock and filled the lifeboats on that side with water. They dropped the anchor on the side away from the dock in an effort to shift enough weight to get the boat back on an even keel. In spite of all their efforts, the wind kept pushing the *Hygiene* further and further over. Rex called to us, "Go sit in the dining salon on the uphill side; we need all the weight we can get on that side." I wasn't sure he was serious.

Shortly after, Gus poked his head in and said, "You better get out on deck and stay on the upper side. There's a possibility we might roll. We don't want anyone trapped."

It did not take us long to get outside! Every time the ship lurched, the dock did too, and it looked as though it would go right along with us if we went over. Soon the wind dropped a bit, and everything held until the *Hygiene* floated again. We breathed a sigh of relief after we moved out to an "unprotected" anchorage and felt the gentle, buoyant roll of the ship through the night.

A minimal number of cases of tuberculosis and venereal disease showed up in this mainly Caucasian and recently immigrated community. While we worked in the clinic, Jessie and Larry went on a search for food. They found half a cow, and Jessie thought she had a pig in addition. His name was Henry.

When the fellows went in to pick up the pig, the young farmer who had promised Henry to Jessie told them with some embarrassment, "Henry looked up at me with such trust, I couldn't kill him. We've been friends for quite a while, and I'm going to keep him around a bit longer."

Jessie said, "He'll probably die of old age." She was able to get 100 pounds each of fresh cabbage, carrots, and potatoes. After our many meals of canned food, they were delicious.

A saying developed on board, "If anything can go wrong, it will in Cook Inlet." Miss Eby, the nursing supervisor from Anchorage, had planned to rendezvous with us several times, but emergencies canceled the meetings. Now she was scheduled to fly from Anchorage to Homer, where we planned to work on Tuesday, but true to form, an emergency arose. One of the townspeople brought a critically ill patient to see the doctor after dinner. Dr. Krusich said it was imperative that the patient be hospitalized in Seldovia as soon as possible.

She sent Gus into town to bring back Larry and the rest of the crew who had gone in that afternoon to check out the bars. Gus found the crew having a high time. Normally they did not drink if they knew they would be traveling, but this was a surprise. Larry told the doctor that he and the crew were not in shape to take the ship out. Dr. Krusich convinced him this was a matter of life and death for the patient, and it was not far.

Larry, in no condition to argue with her, said, "Susie, you come up on the bridge and give me a hand. Kitty, get the coffee going and see that everyone drinks it." Gus had not been uptown, so he was all right on the engines. Larry went over the course and headings with me, then rang the bells for Gus in the engine room, and the ship came to life. Except for having to leave their party, the crew was feeling no pain as they cast off. Larry was sitting hunched over the chart table, asking me what my headings were as we pulled out into the channel. So far, all was running smoothly, but the *Hygiene* was still in the shelter of Kachemak Bay.

Kitty came up to the bridge with a cup of coffee for Larry and said that all below were having a mug-up, and Jessie was serving pie. Just about then the *Hygiene* came out into the tides and wind of Cook Inlet and began plunging and beating in the pitch dark. This was scary enough when everyone was operating at full capacity, but it was terrifying when the captain and the crew were definitely not in complete control. Larry was sobering up fast. The next hurdle was to get enough of the crew in shape to make the landing and tie up in Seldovia.

Kitty and I both were scared and worried. She stayed with me on the bridge, and we kept Larry talking and checking on course headings. Soon, much to our relief, the lights of Seldovia began to appear. One by one, crew members came up to the pilot house in a more or less sober state. Dr. Krusich stayed with her patient and later admitted she had second thoughts about the hazards she had forced on the ship and crew, even though her patient desperately needed hospital care.

Miss Eby then arrived in Homer as scheduled, but we were in Seldovia. By the time she found a flight to Seldovia, we had moved to Port Graham, where we had gone to finish X-raying. There she finally caught up with us.

Extreme cold prevented us from completing our program. Pipes froze on the ship, and it was hard to keep warm. We all had different systems for fending off the cold. After conferring with several Natives, I assembled a comfortable outfit. It consisted of long woollies under jeans plus a wool sweater over a wool shirt. Heavy wool socks under fur mukluks lined with thick felt insoles kept my feet warm. By adding a wool-lined windproof jacket with a hood, a wool cap, scarf, and mittens under some large beaded moosehide mitts, I did not feel the biting wind and snow as I went back and forth from ship to shore.

Dr. Krusich swore by her big fur coat that completely covered her. Kitty, as always, looked very trim and professional in her navy blue wool slacks, long navy blue coat, and her jaunty navy blue nurse's hat. No one could see the layers underneath that rounded her figure.

Miss Eby brought a fresh perspective to our program and personnel problems. Dr. Krusich had stubbornly persisted in trying to follow a schedule set up in the Juneau office, where no one had the knowledge to predict or even imagine the conditions the *Hygiene* would encounter. Miss Eby's complimentary remarks and reassurance undoubtedly helped convince Dr. Krusich that we would gain nothing by going farther into Cook Inlet during the winter months. It was foolhardy and a waste of time that could be better used elsewhere. Dr. Krusich finally, although reluctantly, agreed to head for Seward and Prince William Sound. Amid our rejoicing at this decision, Gus warned, "We still have to cross the Gulf, and we don't have any business being out there this time of year. Terrible storms can blow up. It's dangerous."

At Port Graham the wind was churning the bay like an eggbeater when the *Hygiene* pulled out for the 150-mile trip to Seward. We snugged down for an unpleasant day of rough weather. Instead, when we reached open water, the sea was like glass, the smoothest traveling we had seen in weeks. The sunshine was bright on snow-capped mountains and hills that reached down to the sparkling water.

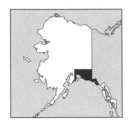

Prince William Sound and Gulf of Alaska

Seward
Saturday, November 16, to Tuesday, November 19

Towering snow-covered mountains embraced Seward, which fit snugly into the narrow valley they formed. Two months earlier we had been impatient to be on our way. Now we had tried the unknown and accomplished nearly all we had set out to do. Although our survey just skimmed the surface, it revealed the complexity of the health and other problems faced by the people of the area. If we could return earlier next year, our constant battle with the weather might be moderated, and we could spend more time working where we were so desperately needed.

Seward represented civilization: docks, water, bars, cars, movies, laundry, and we hoped, mail. Jessie thought that because the town was a major port, it might bring an end to food shortages, but the shipping strike had indeed affected Seward. Here, too, the shelves in the stores were almost bare. Only families with babies could buy canned milk. The TB sanitarium had used all its food supplies and was shipping food in by air to feed the patients. Jessie had enough odds and ends to scrape by, although she was worrying about Thanksgiving. That worry was solved when a storeowner kindly donated one of his own frozen turkeys to the ship.

We became aware of the significance of transportation after we observed the total dependence of the isolated villages on the vagaries and exorbitant rates of the one major steamship company. Bitterness against the Alaska Steamship Line abounded, particularly in Seldovia and Homer. Unreasonable freight rates and the inability of the freighters to deliver supplies during the short summer working period were strangling these burgeoning communities. Their answer was to push for roads to connect them to Anchorage.

Two crew members left us at Seward. One was Chickie, the mascot. She had grown from a three-pound ball of fur to a bouncing, bounding, 13-pound lovable nuisance who happily trailed me around the deck, replenishing her puppy piles as fast as I removed them. When the Greens, managers of the Jessie Lee Home, heard a canine orphan was looking for a home, they welcomed her, as they needed more dogs to play with the children. Chickie was delighted with the arrangement. She had plenty of room to roam about and, above all, dirt to dig in. My life became lonelier but certainly much simpler.

We also lost Bill, the mess boy. His parents were so glad to have him safely back and hear about his experiences that they invited us for dinner. Kitty and I

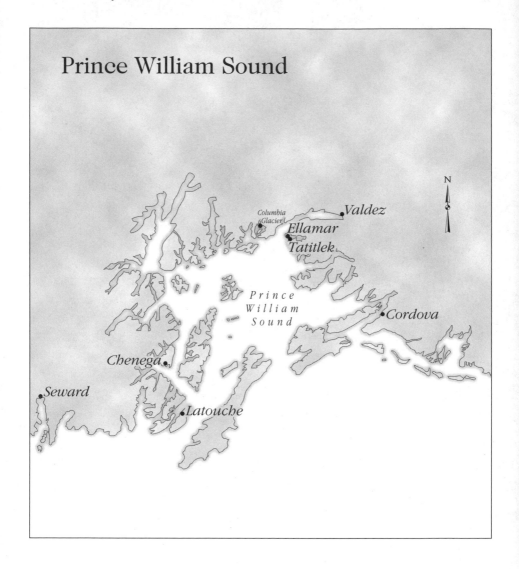

Prince William Sound

Prince William Sound was similar to Southeast Alaska with its protected waters and numerous islands surrounded by glaciers and
mountains. It differed mainly in having colder winter temperatures and
few tourists. The Natives were Eskimos and because they had been in
contact with white Alaskans for several generations, most of the people
spoke English and had some access to medical care, although they lived
in scattered villages. Valdez and Cordova were the largest towns and
had predominantly white populations.

accepted their invitation and thoroughly enjoyed being with these kind people. Following dinner, we attended an adult Sunday school class held at the Greens' home. After an evening of stimulating discussion centering on the topic "What is a Christian?" we realized what a limited field our conversations on the ship had covered. It was inspiring to talk about something other than the ship, our shipmates, and work.

The doctor and some of the crew had headed uptown early in the evening, and after stopping at a few bars, they never gave the Greens' dinner another thought. Even though Kitty and I were hearty eaters, we could not make a dent in a meal prepared for twelve. We were embarrassed by our shipmates' lack of courtesy.

From the heights to the depths! When we arrived back at the ship, a reporter from *Coronet* magazine was waiting to see Dr. Krusich. She planned to do an article on the *Hygiene*, complete with photos. The evening on the town had turned into a full-fledged binge, however, and the crew members who had accompanied the doctor folded her up and sneaked her past the reporter to her stateroom to sleep it off. All was quiet below, but topside, the crew was exploding in a most unethical manner to the reporter, discussing the bickering that had gone on between the doctor and the captain. Even though some of them had obviously been drinking they complained that the doctor had a problem with alcohol. Kitty and I were disgusted, and quietly slipped into our staterooms.

Kitty wrote to Dorothy Whitney, the nursing director, that she did not think she could complete the trip. Despite her belief in the *Hygiene* and the people we were serving, she did not want her name to be associated with this riffraff. Cooling down following a walk in the brisk midnight air, she knocked on my door, and we had a long talk, trying to understand what caused this behavior. We decided that what went on in the *Hygiene's* crew was a reflection of the general Alaskan culture and life in most communities. I prevailed on Kitty to stick it out, at least until the end of this trip.

Seward was the temporary site of the Eklutna School, which was maintained by the Alaska Native Service. The high school students toured the Hygiene while we were in port, and they promised to build a miniature TB isolation unit similar to the maternity demonstration unit Kitty had made. Miss Jund, the health educator, had prepared a set of studies on TB that had aroused the students' interest. Hers was one of the first attempts to prepare health literature in Alaska for Alaskans.

We were disappointed to find that no mail had been been forwarded from Juneau, although we were getting used to being forgotten. At this point, we all needed paychecks.

Latouche and Chenega
Tuesday, November 19, to Friday, November 22

Past tree-covered islands, waterfalls, white clouds, and blue skies mirrored in the calm waters, we sailed to Latouche, once a prosperous copper mine. Where hundreds had lived, now 30 people eked out a living in the tiny ghost town of rusting machinery, tumble-down homes, and sagging boardwalks. We finished our work in Latouche in one afternoon.

Our next stop, Chenega, was a picturesque Native town. In one direction, snowcapped peaks thrust toward the gray sky as it spit snow. In the other direction, a co-op store, a church, a boat shop, and log cabins with smoke rising from their chimneys stretched along the beach of the protected bay. The school, atop a hill guarding the village below, glowed in the occasional rays of the winter sun.

Kitty and I stood on the deck waiting for the usual buzz of an outboard motor. We heard nothing but an occasional duck call. Suddenly I gripped Kitty's arm, "Look, a kayak!" There it was—a slim, elegant craft propelled through the icy waters by men with single-bladed paddles. I was beside myself. I had read and re-lived Baranof's travels around Kodiak Island in these fragile skin boats. I had imagined myself in one of the fleets of tiny kayaks paddling across the Gulf of Alaska to Sitka on a fur hunting expedition. Here was one being used as transportation. I could hardly wait for the paddlers, who turned out to be the schoolteacher and a lay priest, to come aboard so I could talk with them.

After the doctor and captain concluded the official business, I cornered the teacher and bombarded him with questions about his kayak. "Is it hard to paddle? Does it tip easily? Are there any more around?"

Laughingly he answered, "Its called a baidarka, and it does feel quite tippy at first, and yes, there are some old ones around."

The germ of an idea was forming in my mind. It would be great to have a light boat to paddle around and explore the shoreline, as Baranof had done. Also, it would be a means to get away from the bickering on the ship.

Hesitantly I asked, "Would there be any possibility of buying one and, if so, do you know how much it would cost?" "Well-uh," he answered, "maybe about $40. I'll have to let you know when you come ashore."

My next task was to convince the captain that the *Hygiene* needed a skin baidarka. I explained that it was a very small boat and would stow nicely on the upper deck next to my bike and—and it wouldn't grow or leave messes as Chickie did.

With narrowed eyes he looked at me and warned, "It doesn't look safe to me, but if you'll promise to be careful, go ahead and give it a try." I felt like hugging him.

That night I had trouble sleeping, thinking of all the adventures I could have in my baidarka. I was undaunted by the dire predictions voiced by my shipmates. "You'll tip over! That water is *cold*, there's ice floating around in it! Who's going to run the X-ray machine?" Elmer joined me in laughing at their concerns. He wanted to share ownership. Handling the baidarka would be a breeze.

The next day when we went ashore, the teacher told Elmer and me that he had found an old but sound baidarka whose owner would sell it for $40. After we paid for it, we walked down to the beach. Elmer was running the outboard, so I was to paddle it to the ship. It looked a lot narrower than I remembered. The next surprise was that I couldn't sit on the bottom but had to kneel, which gave me an unstable feeling. With shipmates and villagers standing around on the beach expecting me to back out, I felt I had to go ahead and try it. Reassuringly, Elmer called out, "We'll stay right behind you in the rowboat." It was about a 10-minute paddle to the ship, and by the time I arrived, I felt a lot more confidence in our new "toy," but my feet and legs were completely numb. It was all I could do to lift myself onto the ship's ladder. Learning to use this 20-foot-long by two-foot-wide three-cockpit craft was going to be more of a challenge than I had anticipated. Shortly after, Elmer and Rex went out in it together, which was far more difficult. Elmer informed me I could buy him out if I wished.

A funeral interrupted our clinic routines one afternoon. From our vantage point on the ship, we saw the picturesque procession of mourners carrying lighted candles and colorful banners.

On the way to Valdez, we passed the Columbia Glacier, fortunately during the few hours of daylight. This four-mile-wide chunk of ice rose 300 feet straight up from the water and extended 40 miles back into the mountains. When I first saw the glacier, I asked Larry, "Is there time to go down and get my camera?" He laughed and replied, "Only about half an hour; you've lost all sense of perspective because the scale is so grand. When we get closer we may see some large chunks of ice drop into the water, it's called calving. They make quite a splash and sometimes large waves."

As the ship drew nearer, our eyes remained on the wall of ice. Anxiously we waited for one of the huge, jagged spires to topple into the water. The surface appeared more and more craggy, and the blue in the fissures more intense as we sailed just below the formidable face that gave the impression of leaning over us. Kitty and I were frightened—it was all so huge and we were so small. Larry blew our horn and shot his gun toward a large cornice, hoping that the sound waves might start something. I was afraid he might start something larger than we could handle.

Valdez
Friday, November 22, to Thursday, November 28

The weather was getting colder every day. Often a scum of ice formed on the saltwater during the night, and the sun was up only three hours. Valdez was about 80 miles from Chenega, but we found an inch of ice on the water at the entrance to Valdez Bay, in contrast to the relatively open water we had just left. The town resembled the front yard of a glacier. November was drawing to a close, and the temperature was 10 degrees below zero. Again we had difficulty securing water, even though we were moored to a good dock. The men had to lay the water hose about a quarter of a mile. It froze first at the metal couplings, so they heated them with blowtorches to keep the water running.

Mrs. Lindley, the public health nurse, had the town organized for our program when we arrived. From Kodiak on, the X-ray surveying was more efficient because Kitty helped take the films. I particularly needed help when an increase in the laboratory work occurred. Kitty had more free time when the itinerant public health nurses did most of the shore work and organized the communities.

Kitty's and my cooperative work relationship not only made the work go faster but strengthened our friendship. We needed each other's support not only in work, but in the ship's social environment. We both considered the ship as our home for the foreseeable future. Kitty particularly had added homey touches, such as soft cushions on the benches in the dining salon, a record player and records, a slide projector and slides, and her knitting bag.

I invested in a ping pong set we could fasten to the table in the dining salon. Our techniques had to be modified because of the rail around the edge of the table and lack of space, but after dinner we had exciting contests, a change from the continuing poker game.

Dr. Whieldon, the Valdez doctor, was particularly pleased to get chest X-rays of his people. In addition to having a dinner party in our honor, he borrowed an old army truck on Sunday and drove us out the highway as far as Keystone Canyon. A small sign proclaimed that this rough dirt track was the Richardson Highway. The narrow strip of road ran north halfway across

Alaska, joining Valdez on the sea to Fairbanks in the central part of the territory. Near the road, we saw a waterfall that had cascaded down a steep rock wall into a narrow box canyon. The water had frozen while the wind was blowing, and green ice had formed in huge bubbles about 30 feet in diameter all the way down the course of the falls.

In Valdez Dr. Krusich gave a lecture on the psychology of children without families. Many Alaskan children were not necessarily orphans, but lived at schools great distances from their families, and were often unable to communicate with them. This would happen more often as children with TB were hospitalized for long periods of time.

The shipping strike had been hard on Valdez. Empty stores made a bleak outlook for any kind of traditional Thanksgiving meal. When we left for Ellamar on Thanksgiving morning, we saw storekeepers unloading emergency supplies, including turkeys, from a relief ship. They were selling the food on the dock as fast as it was unloaded, and the people carried it directly home for their holiday celebrations.

Ellamar and Tatitlek
Thursday, November 28, to Sunday, December 1

Earlier we had hoped to spend Thanksgiving in the big city of Anchorage, but now not one of us would have traded where we were for Cook Inlet and Anchorage at this time of year. Jessie served us a delicious turkey dinner with all the trimmings in the small village of Ellamar in Prince William Sound. We were thankful to be alive, and to have such a caring person as Jessie, who had squirreled away the goodies for our Thanksgiving under the most difficult conditions.

Ellamar was only 15 miles from Valdez, but the temperature was 15 degrees warmer. Tatitlek, a neighboring small village, was only one mile away. Our program went on at a great pace. It was nearly December, and we looked forward to getting across the Gulf and to Juneau for Christmas, so weekends were like all other workdays.

One afternoon Gus and Rex asked some children if there were any lakes around. They said, "Yes, but you have to cut a hole in the ice to catch fish." The men got their rods and the fire ax and walked with the children to a small lake about halfway between the villages. They chopped several 18-inch-deep holes through the ice, and their efforts were rewarded with enough trout to feed us all.

Cordova
Monday, December 2, to Monday, December 9

Cordova was our last stop on Prince William Sound. Dr. Krusich believed the survey there was nearly perfect. She credited the excellent organization of the town to Betty Little Hodge, a territorial public health nurse, who had arrived only two weeks previously. We X-rayed 1088 Cordovans in three days without any mishaps.

After working hours various residents entertained us. One evening an oldtimer invited us to see his slides of the countryside. He was full of stories about the old days, and he told us of the Cordova Coal Party. In the early 1900s Alaskans around Cordova were paying $11 to $12 a ton for inadequate amounts of imported coal. They were angry, knowing coal fields with a better grade of coal surrounded them and would have cost one fourth the price. The area had been set aside as a national forest, and attempts to make even minor changes had been blocked by legislative inaction over a period of years. Thus the coal at their doorstep was forbidden to them.

One of the Cordovans suggested they have their own version of a Boston Tea Party. The idea caught on, and 300 angry citizens went to the Alaska Steamship dock where a freighter carrying coal from Canada was tied up. The crowd shoveled several tons of coal into the bay. Fortunately, no violence occurred. Unfortunately, Congress took no action, and the Alaskan coal industry did not develop.

During the same period, overdevelopment of salmon fishing on the Copper River had practically wiped out the fishery. Canneries had been located as far as 100 miles up the river, over the protests of the Alaskans of the area. They could see what was happening to the fish runs, and they wanted the river closed to fishing. The river was not closed because representatives of the large canneries dominated the U.S. Department of Commerce, which was supposed to be protecting the salmon runs.

The stories and frustrations of these oldtime Alaskans made us aware of how our government had ignored, abused, and exploited the Territory and its resources. It was evident that Alaska had never been governed for the benefit of Alaskans, but rather for the benefit of those who had the political power to exploit her for their own individual and corporate gains. Many of these oldtimers, and newcomers as well, were working toward statehood.

At last the good news everyone had been waiting for came through: The shipping strike was over! These people had looked forward to a very bleak Christmas, but now relief and rejoicing were everywhere. Supplies would soon be coming north again, hopefully in time for the holidays.

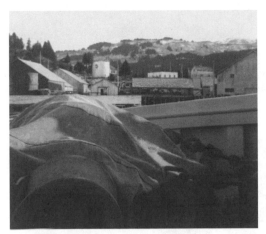
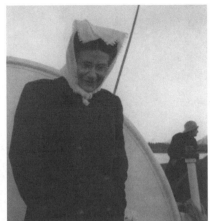
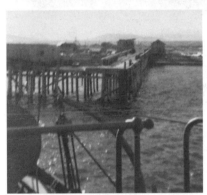
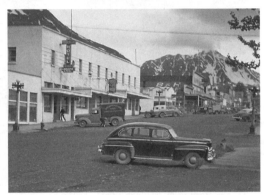
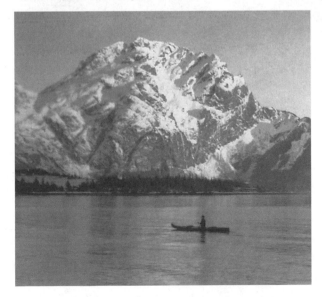
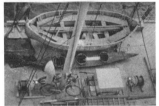

Top: left, Seldovia;
right, Jakie.
Middle: left, Homer;
right, Seward.
Bottom: left, baidarka in
Prince William Sound;
right, baidarka on
upper deck.

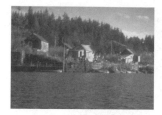

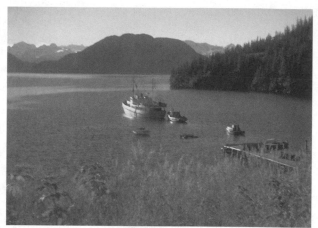

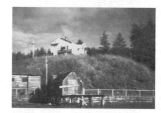

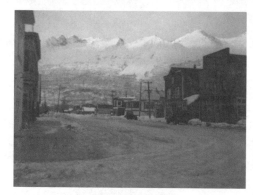

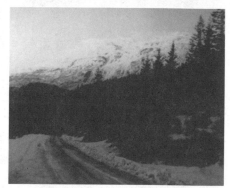

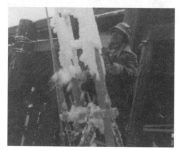

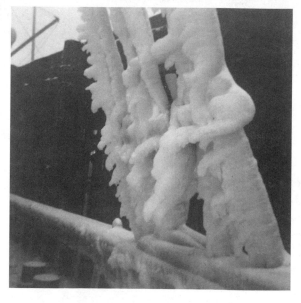

Top: left, two views of Chenega; *right, Hygiene* from Chenega.
Middle: left, Valdez; *right,* Richardson Highway.
Bottom: icy rigging.

Triumphantly we took the last X-ray, finished the last conference, and packed all our equipment for travel across the open ocean to Yakutat. But this was December—the good weather ended, and a blizzard struck. The Gulf of Alaska was preparing to show its other side. We waited two days in Cordova for the storm to end. Then we received a telegram from the Juneau office saying, "Skip Yakutat; come directly to Juneau." That meant after a 30-hour run across the gulf and a few more hours in sheltered waters, we would arrive in Juneau, an event we eagerly anticipated. But that was not to be.

Cordova to Yakutat
Monday, December 9, to Saturday, December 14

When we left the protection of Prince William Sound, the violent temper of the gulf in winter hit us. Wind-driven spray and waves washed over the entire ship. This was nothing new, and we settled down for a day of unpleasant traveling. Pleasant thoughts of the Christmas holiday that lay ahead filled our minds. Kitty and I had reservations on a flight to Pennsylvania and New York on December 19, 10 days away. The timing seemed to be good.

On our second day out, the wind picked up. The sea became even rougher as we approached the St. Elias Range with its vast icefields and glaciers that had been so beautiful on the way north. Now a new element, low temperature, added to the wind and waves. The cold caused every drop of water that hit the *Hygiene* to freeze on her. Ice coated the sides of the pilot house and its windows, making it impossible to see out.

Larry sent Rex to the clinic for a small heater to melt a peephole for the person at the wheel. Rex was gone longer than we expected. He returned visibly shaken, saying, "That damn deck is covered with ice. I thought I'd had it when one of those waves hit me. I almost went over the rail—it's covered with ice too!" Larry said to pass the word around for everyone to remain indoors. Kitty was trapped in her stateroom, and I was trapped out of mine, which was all right with me. I was much less afraid in dangerous situations if I had a job to do and knew what was happening.

I spent the time on the bridge, where they needed an extra hand to hold the electric heater against the window to clear peepholes for the helmsman to look through, and to free the compass when the deeper rolls caused it to stick in the gimbals. The next day I discovered large bruises on both my hips from being wedged between the compass stand and the bulkhead.

In a letter to her father Kitty wrote:

Cordova to Yakutat was a sad, sad story. It stormed and it iced—we rolled and we pitched—and I heaved and I heaved. Drawers fell out, things spilled, and my room was a shambles. I guess it seemed bad 'cause it was a thirty-two hour stretch of rough water. We just had to face it and keep going until we reached Yakutat, the only safe place to anchor along the whole coastline.

The boys said if we had taken much more ice, we'd have been in real danger. Apparently icing is one thing no ship can take long, 'cause they get top-heavy and roll right over. The Gulf is a graveyard for several such ships.

Laden with ice, we pulled into Yakutat in the late afternoon of December 11. The weather was too severe for us to continue south across the Gulf. Pale people began to appear on deck, gazing in wonder at and photographing our ice-shrouded ship.

Jessie, coming up from her bunk, said, "I'll cook up some hamburgers."

The skipper replied, "You will like hell. You'll fry up those steaks we bought in Cordova. We haven't had a meal since we left there."

"Amen," the crew agreed.

Despite the telegram from Juneau, we carried on with the original program for the next three days while we waited for a break in the weather. Miss Simons, the Alaska Native Service nurse, and the schoolteachers helped us organize the village. The residents were not at their best because their water supply had been frozen for two weeks. While we waited and worked, we prayed for the temperature and wind to moderate.

Yakutat to Juneau
Saturday, December 14, to Thursday, December 19

December 14 brought a "so-so" weather forecast, and we set out for Juneau about 4 p.m. Proud to have completed the program, we expected to be in Juneau on December 15. Rex kidded Steve, a Catholic, that we would not get to Juneau in time for him to go to church. Steve allowed as how he would probably pray enough by the time we reached our destination to make up for it. He wasn't kidding!

When we rounded Ocean Cape, the Gulf of Alaska again hit us with its winter rage. Every drop of water froze on the ship. The rigging cables, normally three-quarters of an inch in diameter, grew to nearly a foot thick. Ice again covered the sides of the ship as high as the pilot house. Because the wind was coming from the starboard quarter, the weight of the ice was double on that side.

After a few hours I hesitantly asked, not wanting to sound timid, "Does anyone else feel like we are awfully alone out here?"

Rex comfortingly said, "This is a seaworthy ship, but a combination of wind and cold can sink the best of them." He then proceeded to tell gloom-and-doom stories of fishing boats that had turned over in ice storms and been lost without a trace.

While I listened to his tales, the *Hygiene* would roll far over to starboard, but instead of righting herself quickly, as she normally did, she would stay there and stay there until, ever so slowly, with tremendous creaking and groaning, the ice-laden, top-heavy hull would begin to stand back up, and I would find myself breathing again for a few moments. Larry had a weather report that conditions should moderate shortly, so he decided to stick it out.

Rex was worried. He went down to the engine room. He wanted Gus to persuade Larry to turn back. Even down there, Gus could tell that the ship was icing badly, but he told Rex to go back up on the bridge where he belonged. Gus did come up to the bridge to hear the next weather report. The forecast had changed drastically. The voice on the radio described a tanker that had been trying to get around Cape Spencer for two days. Now they no longer expected any improvement for 12 hours. Neither Gus nor Larry liked the feel of the ship, and after a brief consultation Larry decided to head back to Yakutat. By turning the ship around, he could build some ice on the other side to balance it.

The ship's rolls were still uneven and drawn out. I found my thoughts nostalgically going back to the safe, crowded Seattle bus on which I had ridden back and forth to work, the busy grocery stores, a quiet warm house, meals at regular times.... Maybe something could be said for routine jobs. After a seemingly endless time, in reality only about three hours, the light indicating the entrance to Yakutat Bay showed. By then the ship's rolls had evened out somewhat, but she still righted herself sluggishly due to the tremendous weight of the ice above the water line.

Again we tied up to the dock in Yakutat. The medical staff and some of the crew began to appear from their bunks. When we climbed out on the dock to look at the ship we could hardly believe what we saw. The entire ship and rigging were sheathed in ice, in places more than a foot thick. In an eerie way it was beautiful and looked like a ghost ship, though we were glad it was not. But soon we were laughing and comparing stories about how we had felt. Ruthie had even put on her life jacket, which would not have helped at all in the icy waters.

Instead of walking the streets of Juneau as we had planned, we were grateful to be alive. The next morning we broke the ice from the ship's sides and rigging with axes, crowbars, and hammers. All, including Dr.

Krusich, took part and enjoyed the hard work. The men shoveled huge piles of ice off the deck. No one wanted a speck of ice left on the ship for the next try at crossing the gulf. All the while, though the sun shone, the temperature did not rise, and the wind continued to blow. We felt very close to one another after sharing the frightening experiences of the last two days. Past disagreements and frustrations seemed to be forgotten.

The MV *Hygiene* returned to Juneau December 19, after completing her first journey across the Gulf of Alaska. We had carried a modern health program to people almost untouched by modern medicine, in an inaccessible area. We had taken nearly 4000 chest X-rays since leaving Juneau on August 29.

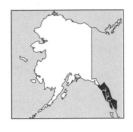

4

Southeast Alaska Revisited

1947

After a much-needed Christmas vacation, Dr. Krusich, Kitty, and I returned to Juneau. Several days of conferences with our department heads and with Dr. Albrecht gave us a broader viewpoint of the overall program. Many changes were underway. The rapid expansion of the Health Department, the money problems, and the politics involved in keeping the Hygiene and other units going and growing were overwhelming.

Juneau
Sunday, January 12, to Thursday, January 16

DR. ALBRECHT TOLD US of his plans to send a mobile screening unit by plane to the interior and the far north. Another was to be installed on the railroad. He had plans for two more ships; one for the Yukon River, and another shallow-draft vessel that would be more suitable for the Bering Sea than the *Hygiene*. The truck unit was already serving the highway. The sanitarium at Seward, when it reached full capacity, would add about 200 hospital beds to the 100 already in use. Another 200 beds would come on line at Sitka when personnel could be found to staff them. The Sanitation Division, Laboratory Division, and Itinerant Public Health Nursing Service were all expanding. Significant amounts of money had been appropriated by the territorial and federal governments to fight tuberculosis.

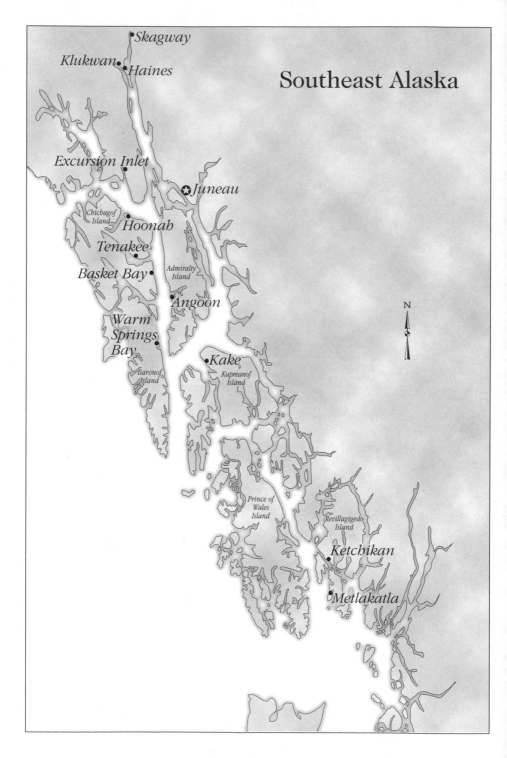

Southeast Alaska

Skagway

Klukwan • Haines

Excursion Inlet

Juneau

Chichagof Island

Hoonah

Tenakee

Basket Bay

Admiralty Island

Angoon

Warm Springs Bay

Baronof Island

Kake

Kupreanof Island

N

Prince of Wales Island

Revillagigedo Island

Ketchikan

Metlakatla

One of Dr. Albrecht's most difficult tasks was to find qualified personnel to fill these new positions. Even more difficult was finding places for them to live. Housing was critical all over Alaska because none had been built during the war, and now high freight rates had created a grave shortage of building materials.

We on the *Hygiene's* medical staff began to see that in this exciting time of dreams, trials, confusion, and rapid growth, it was understandable that the small office force in Juneau might be so busy they could forget to send mail or to keep a radio schedule. The *Hygiene* was far away, and many more immediate pressures bore on them. A constant state of crisis prevailed.

On the other hand, we were able to give the personnel of the health department a better understanding of the problems we faced with weather and transporting patients between the ship and shore. Kitty and Dr. Krusich emphasized the need for teaching materials that people lacking any knowledge of infection or sanitation could understand. We weren't sure the departmental staff adequately comprehended how difficult it was for the doctor and Kitty to tell people who were very ill and spoke little English that they knew they were sick, but we couldn't help them just now. Getting these patients into a sanitarium was essential for two reasons: to prevent further spread of disease in the crowded living quarters and, just as important, to let the Native people know we were doing something to help them.

Dr. Krusich explained that health education was essential, particularly in the isolated communities. She also pointed out that in order to get any kind of cooperation at our stops, the ship's doctor had to take care of immediate health problems before tackling the X-ray survey and other long-range projects.

Dr. Krusich, Kitty, and I were elated at Dr. Albrecht's decision to have the *Hygiene* spend a month in each of the five largest villages in Southeast Alaska. At least in this area, we would have time to properly attend to medical problems and education. An equally important benefit emerged: we could refer active cases to the new TB hospital opening in Sitka. Hope replaced the feeling of despair that had pervaded our program on the westward trip. After our somewhat harrowing experiences on that trip, we were happy to hear the *Hygiene* would be in the protected waters of Southeast Alaska for the winter. Summer months were the proper time for us to meet the challenges offered by a survey of the Eskimo villages surrounding the Bering Sea.

Jessie, Gus, and Rex had stayed on the ship during Christmas vacation. The fellows built and painted new cupboards and shelves. Kitty was thrilled to find a kneehole desk in her stateroom. No longer would she have to study and write curled up like a pretzel on her bunk.

Hoonah
Thursday, January 16, to Sunday, February 16

Following the now-familiar routine of filling the empty crew positions and loading supplies, we left Juneau at 8 a.m. and covered the 80 miles to Hoonah by that afternoon. A town less than a day's travel away seemed almost next door, but in midwinter, we were to find, even the protected waters of Southeast Alaska could isolate one village from another.

When we turned off Icy Strait into Hoonah Bay, we could see, even from a distance, that this community was different. Instead of a string of irregularly spaced, variously sized and sunbleached houses that fit into the landscape, these houses looked like intruders. Nearly identical buildings formed regular street patterns. All were the same style, the only difference being that some were painted and others were weathered.

We learned later that in the late 1930s most of Hoonah had burned to the ground. The residents crowded into the remaining homes or lived in tents for several years until the Bureau of Indian Affairs built houses under the auspices of the Federal Housing Act. The dwellings, reasonably priced at $3000, were sold to the Indians for $450 down, with the balance to be paid off in 20 years. Good-looking boats tied up at the docks and anchored in the bay gave this community an appearance of prosperity.

Miss Bock, the nurse, and Mayor Harry Douglas met us at the dock. Harry told us a little about the town. He was proud of the fact that in the previous year it had become one of the few incorporated Native towns in Alaska. This meant that individuals could own town lots and tax themselves for local improvements, he explained. At the moment the town was financially embarrassed, but when the residents had collected some taxes, they planned to improve their waterworks, electric plant, and dock. He hoped to avoid the years of waiting if they depended on the federal government to do it.

Our first impression, given by the outspoken younger people, was that the mayor was doing a fine job, but it did not take long to discover that the town had several factions. All were proud of their Tlingit blood, and the older generation was particularly anxious to hold on to their culture. They thought that young couples should be moving into the clan houses rather than buying their own homes. All factions were conscious, however, that Hoonah could become a model for other villages to follow, and that the rest of Alaska was watching them.

Harry officially welcomed us to the town. He proudly explained that an eight-piece band provided music for a dance every Saturday night, a movie house showed films at regular intervals, and the Civilian Conservation Corps had built a ski trail and shelter a mile and a half south of town. Three stores competed for the business of the locals and the summer fishing crowd. He pointed out it was a dry town because the citizens had voted against liquor being sold there. He hoped we would enjoy our stay.

Then Dr. Krusich described our program. We would base the schedule on family units rather than offering separate clinics for TB, children, and so forth. We would give thorough physical exams to everyone and allow time for follow-up treatments on all those with health problems. She had scheduled a general clinic for every Friday. The medical staff would offer instruction on a number of public health topics, using movies and slide shows. Finally, we would post a schedule of events weekly in each store and on the *Hygiene*. We hoped to get 100 percent coverage of the town.

As I sat listening to the plans, my mind flashed back to Kodiak Island and Cook Inlet and the hours we had wasted waiting for weather. Of working day and night when the weather was good, and of being stuck on board unable to work or go ashore for a change of scene when it was bad. Now we could plan ahead. We would be working eight hours a day and would have Saturday afternoons and Sundays off. We were tied to a dock. People could come aboard when they were scheduled, and we could go ashore. It brought home to me how I had taken these everyday conveniences for granted until I did not have them.

One day Kitty was presenting a slide show on the home care of TB. The actors in the show were Indians and friends of the villagers. While Kitty was giving the narration that accompanied the pictures, she unconsciously threw herself into the different parts so earnestly that she was speaking with a Tlingit accent. Gus and Rex were afraid the Natives would take offense, but instead it amused them, and they were more friendly than ever.

The first few days in Hoonah, I X-rayed, Kitty drew blood samples, and Dr. Krusich gave talks to an active town council, the Alaska Native Brotherhood, and the Alaska Native Sisterhood. The audience asked intelligent questions, especially about TB, which pleased the doctor. These village leaders wanted to help and offered to bring in neighbors who they knew should be seen but did not come when scheduled. This kind of local participation was invaluable.

Saturday afternoon Kitty and I put on our skis and followed a trail along the shore to look for the ski area. We found the hill, a small cleared slope in the woods with a shelter at the bottom. A large outdoor fireplace and stove suggested the possibility for a Sunday cookout in the snow. Sure enough, Sunday afternoon seven other people from the *Hygiene* trudged the mile and a half to the shelter carrying hot dogs, buns, and soup. Rex built a roaring fire, and we took turns on the two pairs of skis, eating and warming up. The snow was deep and soft, so it did not matter that few of the group had ever been on skis before.

On Monday the clinic routines started. On Tuesday, word came from Juneau that a visiting doctor and his nurse would be staying on board for a few days. They were working on an experimental vaccine to prevent TB, and we were to help them in any way we could.

Dr. Krusich sputtered, "There goes our program," and I for once agreed with her.

The next morning the visitors arrived. I looked at the visiting doctor and he looked at me.

"Colonel Aronson!" I exclaimed, while he was saying "Susan Hull, what are you doing here?"

I had worked for him for two years at Fort Lewis near Tacoma, Washington, during the war. This warm, jolly man was so different from the formal officer I had been somewhat in awe of at the Fort.

While the doctors were making plans to coordinate their work over the usual "mug-up" in the galley, Dr. Aronson started to tell us about the controversy over the use of BCG. Jessie hesitantly asked, "Could you explain what BCG is?"

He grinned, pointed a finger at me and said, "Susan, you should be able to do that."

"Well, let's see, B stands for Bacillus, and C and G stand for Calmette and Guerin, they were Frenchmen, and quite a while back they fooled around with a TB bug and changed it so that when people were inoculated with it they became immune. Sort of like a smallpox vaccination. But I'm not sure what the controversy is about."

Dr. Aronson took over. "This vaccine has been used successfully all around the world—Norway, Denmark, Russia, Japan—since about 1927...."

Kitty and I spoke at once; "Why can't we use it here?"

Dr. Aronson replied, "That's exactly what we're working on. The problem is that no one has done a study with adequate controls to prove the effectiveness of BCG to the satisfaction of the U.S. Public Health Service." He continued, "In 1935 I started an experiment to do this. We vaccinated Natives in 12 villages up here. First we had to find those who did not have the disease. Then half were vaccinated and the other half were given a placebo. We checked these people regularly until the war interrupted our program in 1941. At that time we found that 40 people in the vaccinated group had developed TB, but in the group inoculated with salt solution 185 cases developed. That is not 100 percent protection, but in an epidemic area such as Alaska, it is worthwhile.

"The opposition to BCG comes from the doctors in the States. Some feel that it prevents discovery of active cases through the use of the tuberculin test. This is true, because everyone inoculated with BCG has a positive tuberculin test, but as you know, there are other ways of diagnosing TB." Here was another case where decisions were made for Alaska by people who were not aware of all the factors involved.

We quickly recognized how valuable BCG could be to Alaska, especially in the remote areas, and we were eager to help his project. Dr. Aronson and Miss Parr, his nurse, brought new life and hope to the program to eradicate tuberculosis. Even Dr. Krusich became enthusiastic and was a cooperative and charming hostess, showing a side of her character we had not seen before.

I learned a great deal working with Miss Parr, a tall angular, down-to-earth, middle-aged lady who had a delightful sense of humor. Involved in the American BCG experiment from the beginning, she had held things together while Dr. Aronson was gone during the war. Living and working under all kinds of primitive conditions, she had developed and recovered from a severe case of radiation sickness due to using improperly shielded X-ray equipment. Her description of the nausea, weakness, loss of hair, and anemia that lasted over a period of months greatly increased my respect for the powerful machine with which I was working. I felt, as did everyone else, that Miss Parr was one of the unsung heroines of the medical profession.

The work for the BCG research study was done within four days and had only slightly interfered with our program. In fact, having an extra doctor and nurse had been quite helpful, especially the day an Indian came in with a badly cut and bleeding hand.

Dr. Aronson recommended that we establish regular clinics to check the ship's personnel. He pointed out that in the crowded, poorly ventilated clinic we constantly were exposed to active cases of TB. From that time on I regularly X-rayed the people working on the ship.

The Hygiene, tied out of the wind, was snug and warm, even though the temperature outside hung around zero, and the snow piled up. On Saturday afternoon, while I skied around the town, I met Mr. Olsen, a Swedish fisherman who had lived in Hoonah for 25 years. He urged me to tell our crew that they should not miss the dance that night because the high-school glee club was going to perform. A large group of us went and enjoyed the program, and we found some local additions to the ski party we had planned for the next day, and also borrowed several pairs of skis.

On Sunday morning the temperature was still zero, and more snow had fallen during the night, but it did not dampen enthusiasm for the ski party and cookout. It was such a pleasure to be able to step out the door and put on skis. One young man named Earl came along with his snowshoes. He gave all of us a chance to try them. Kitty, who had never tried skiing until she came to Hoonah, said it was the most fun she had ever had doing anything athletic. Mr. Olsen came out and showed us how they skied in the old country with one pole between the legs. Jessie, with many helpers, cooked a marvelous dinner over the roaring fire in the shelter.

When we returned, Miss Bock invited us in to her cozy, warm house to drink a big pot of hot chocolate she had made. She commented, "I hope our people can see how much fun you are having—even in bad weather. They need this type of recreation in the winter. It would be so good for the younger people if they had a recreation director to get them out."

On Tuesday a very sick woman came in needing hospitalization. Larry got through to Juneau on the radio and asked for an emergency plane to take her to the hospital, but the plane didn't come for a long time. Finally we heard and then saw it flying just above the water. When the pilot, Shell Simmons, one of the best in Alaska, stepped out he said, "Whew, that was rough. Nothing but a critically ill person would have brought me. It's so cold the water froze on my floats, and I couldn't gain any altitude. Alaska Coastal has canceled all flights."

That explained why there had not been any planes the last few days. The extremely cold weather was most unusual for the area. Saltwater was freezing in the shallows, and where it remained liquid, the water was so much warmer than the air that it steamed like a bathtub.

Two days later the mail boat *Estebeth* came in laden with ice. After the crew chopped it off, Dr. Aronson and Miss Parr boarded, hoping to reach Angoon. After a week's delay, they were eager to get on with their work. Regretfully we said good-bye. They had been a great addition to shipboard life.

That afternoon I was busy working in the lab when who should appear but Miss Parr. In answer to my puzzled look, she said, "When we rounded the point into Icy Strait, the waves were washing over us and we were icing down so fast that the captain turned back and ran for shelter." I knew exactly what she meant.

Again the weary *Estebeth* crew chopped away ice in preparation for an early start in the morning. Again they said good-bye. And again, the *Estebeth* returned covered with ice, still carrying Dr. Aronson and Miss Parr. They had

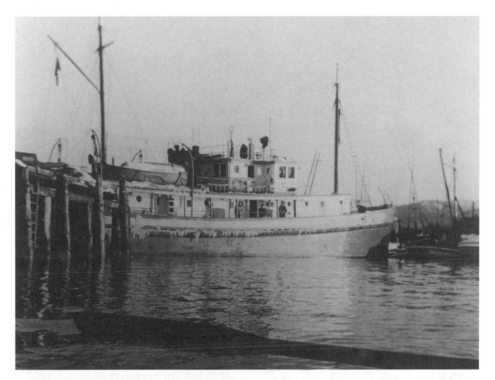

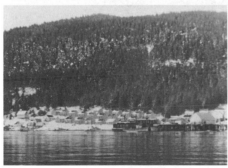

Top: Hygiene in Hoonah.
Above: Hoonah.
Right: Ed, Jim, Capt. Crosby,
and Wayne.

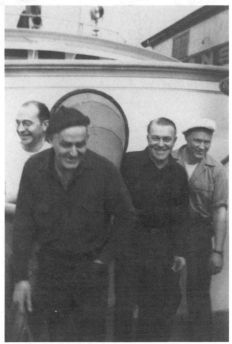

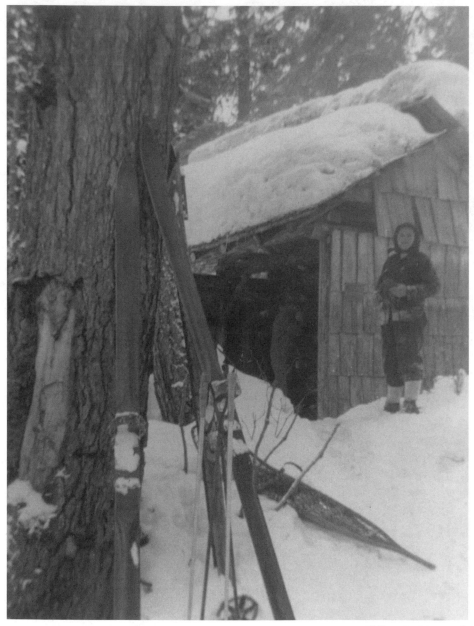

Skiing in Hoonah

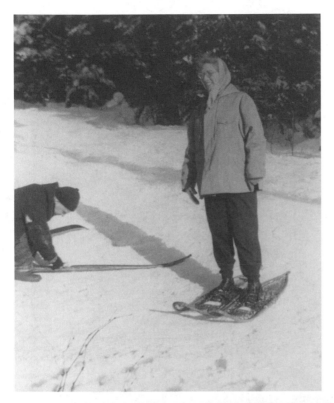

Left: Susie
Below: Morris and Meg

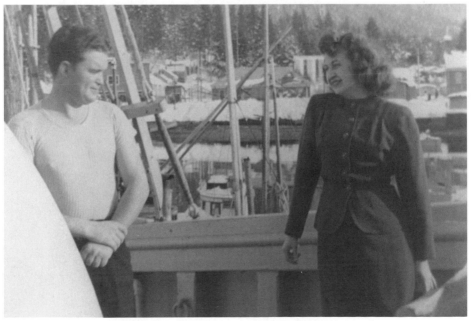

made it to Chatham Strait and had a long enough period of rolling around for Miss Parr to get really seasick. Even the ebullient Dr. Aronson was getting discouraged as the crew chopped ice for the third time. Weather conditions remained the same for two more days, and the *Estebeth* waited. Finally, five days after their first departure, the temperature moderated slightly and they were able to reach Angoon, only 60 miles away.

Dr. Krusich was very amusing during this period. While Dr. Aronson was around she was on her best behavior and was most gracious and entertaining. When he left she would heave a sigh of relief and become her old, brusque self. Then he would return, and again she would become a charming hostess. After the third character change, even she saw the humor of the situation.

The month that some had dreaded as being a long time to stay in a place like Hoonah was flying by. We had found friends and activities of interest. The townspeople enjoyed movies, even health movies. The attendance at the TB movie was unusually good because it was advertised "For adults only." Seating space and not movie content was the real reason for the restriction to adults. In turn, we appreciated the town's theater.

Our friend Mr. Olsen was a frequent visitor, and one Sunday after church he took Kitty and me on a ski trip to the Icy Strait Cannery. It was around the point from the bay where the *Hygiene* was docked. On the way we passed a Russian cemetery with very ornate tombstones.

On the end of the point a small house, open on the side facing the water, marked the grave of an early Indian chief. Mr. Olsen said another chief was buried in a house just like it on the point forming the other side of the entrance to the bay. Many of the Natives still believed the two chiefs were standing watch to keep evil spirits from coming into the town.

The cannery, closed in the winter, was a cold and ugly place. Mr. Olsen lamented that the fishing was poorer every year. The local fishermen blamed this on the fish traps that they had opposed for years. He explained that most of the traps belonged to companies that were not Alaskan-owned and did not even pay property taxes. The Alaskans predicted that these companies would take all the fish and then leave them with nothing. They were bitter about the situation, as all legislation passed favored the canneries. The pressure for statehood was popping up everywhere, and it was easy to understand.

Employment in the canneries was also a sore point, because most employees were brought in from the States, and Alaskans were only hired in emergencies. After the complaints we had heard in Cook Inlet and Prince William Sound about the management of the fishery industry, we were beginning to suspect that the stories we had heard of the robberies of fish traps by local fishermen were nothing compared to the grandiose robberies the canneries had perpetrated in Alaska.

One Sunday morning Kitty, Meg (our latest secretary who had come aboard in Juneau), and I left the ship to attend the Presbyterian church but were detoured to the Russian Orthodox church because the Presbyterians were not having a service that morning. Kitty and I had been in the Russian Orthodox church at Belkofsky, but this was the first service we had experienced. It was most unusual. Everyone stood the entire two-and-a-half hours, and they did not stand in one place, but moved about freely. The priest spoke in Russian or Tlingit, we could not decide which. The lay reader read from the Bible in English. The congregation's chants, church robes, and the altar were beautiful.

We had to close our eyes when the entire congregation kissed the same cross and drank from the same goblet. By this time we knew that some of these people were active cases of TB. We prayed the sacredness of the act would kill the germs.

A remarkable number of Hoonah's residents were overweight, so Kitty, with Dr. Krusich's approval, started a nutrition class. The night before the class started, Kitty had seconds of everything on the dinner table, excusing herself because she was going on a diet with her class, and this would be her last good meal. The turnout for Kitty's diet classes was discouragingly small. Many adults came in later, however, to ask for the printed reducing diets.

The tremendous number of overweight people amazed Dr. Krusich. She wrote in her report, "If this obesity problem persists in other Southeastern towns, we should include it with our medical clinic and give these people complete physical examinations to try to determine if there is any physical factor in their being overweight. I think too, it might be wise to try some amphetamine sulphate to control appetites. Obesity should not be treated lightly. It is now considered one of the important factors in causes of death."

The doctor studied the eating habits of the people in Hoonah. She reported that on the average they ate three eggs a week, citrus fruits once or twice a week, very few yellow or green vegetables, and much macaroni, rice, cereals, and brown beans. Milk was generally made into cocoa. They made little use of wild greens and had no gardens.

One morning the flag at the post office was flying at half mast. When Miss Bock came to the ship Kitty asked "Who died? We didn't hear about anything on the radio."

"It was a former chief," Miss Bock replied. "He was very old." Later Harry Douglas came to the ship to invite us to the funeral on Friday afternoon. He warned that the village would be in mourning for the next week, and all social activities would be canceled. When Friday came, we made every effort to finish the clinics early, but it was one of those days that could not be hurried. We missed the first part of the funeral and the singing, but arrived in time to hear a band of about 15 oldtimers playing a dirge. They played well, and we could feel their sorrow. Practically the entire village was packed into the little church.

After the service, the pallbearers placed the coffin on a sled and pulled it the length of the town. The band accompanied it and had plenty of opportunity to play all the funeral marches they knew. The pallbearers then loaded the coffin onto a couple of small fishing boats tied together and the procession went to Graveyard Island, directly across the bay from town.

Rex borrowed a rowboat, and he, Meg, and I rowed over to the island, but we did not go ashore. Large, brightly colored paper flowers the townspeople had made covered the casket. The relatives carried large bouquets of paper flowers. Miss Bock told Kitty that in a year the clan would hold a potlatch, and all who gave anything—music, gravedigging, flowers, or transportation—would receive money. Something like $4000 to $5000 would exchange hands. She said some of the villagers thought, and many whites would agree, that too much was made over the dead and not enough over the living.

Miss Bock explained that they held the potlatch feast so the departed's spirit would be strong enough to enter and live in a future newborn. This also explained why they did not punish little children when they misbehaved, because it would mean punishing the spirit of an elder who had died, and that would show a lack of respect.

The last week we spent in Hoonah, we tied up the loose ends at work and said farewell to our new friends. An unplanned activity interrupted our full schedule. The temperature had moderated several days earlier, but it was not until Monday morning that the ice floes that had formed in the shallow bays broke loose. Their advance threatened the dock and the Hygiene. The men of the village and the Hygiene broke the ice with pickaxes into manageable-size pieces and disengaged them from the pilings so they could drift into open water. Only after they had maneuvered the floes around the dock could we continue the clinic work.

Social activities reached a peak during the last few days. The grand finale was a wedding followed by a formal dance. Dr. Krusich and I had to miss the wedding and reception because just as we were leaving to attend the ceremony, a little girl with a broken elbow was carried aboard. From the ship I was able later to get a glimpse of the bridal party as they walked down the path from the church to their house. The bride had on a long white dress with a six-foot train; three bridesmaids and a flower girl in long, very bright pink dresses followed her. Kitty told us that the bridal party was half an hour late for the ceremony, but the guests accepted this as normal.

The dance was a formal affair, and many of the ladies wore long dresses. The mayor opened the festivities by asking the bride to dance, and the bridegroom danced with the mayor's wife. The guests watched the two couples through the first dance, and then all joined in the next waltz.

Later that evening as we walked back to the ship, I told Kitty that I found it hard to believe I could be so genuinely sorry to leave a small Indian village in Alaska. The people, both Indian and white, had welcomed us so hospitably, cooperated in the work, and included us in their village activities so graciously. We both knew this was a village we would not forget.

Some of the findings and recommendations in Dr. Krusich's report on Hoonah gave an in-depth look at the health picture at that time:

> We took 517 four-by-five X-rays and found 44 with tuberculosis. Out of the 250 blood samples drawn for Kahns, 16 were positive.
>
> Through diet studies done in the school, the nutritional status of the children seems to be above average. On physical examinations, leaving out the bad teeth that seem to be endemic in Alaska, the children seem to be well cared for on the whole. It would be an excellent service if the Territorial Department of Health could send a medical officer once a month to these nearby villages to conduct infant, preschool, and prenatal clinics. A great deal of generalized health education could be put out in such clinics.
>
> In the field of health education it has seemed that too frequently we stick by established methods that have not only failed elsewhere but fail in the native villages.... It is useless to blame a community for their lack of interest in some service that we feel valuable. It is our business to develop a health education program that will appeal to our clientele. Inasmuch as people in these Native villages enjoy movies a great deal, I think it would be wise to build our health education around movies. We could then make an opportunity for the audience to ask questions and participate in the program.
>
> This community needs regular medical care, and I have suggested to the local council that they get together with the surrounding villages and see if it

would be possible under some sort of insurance plan to contract with a physician to make scheduled visits. I have also suggested that they request of the Territorial Health Department certain regular public health services, and sanitary inspections.

Excursion Inlet
Sunday, February 16, to Tuesday, February 18

Low fog surrounded us when we left Hoonah early Sunday morning on the two-hour run to Excursion Inlet. Tips of mountains glowed in the sunlight high above us. What kind of craggy cliffs or tree-lined shores lay between was anyone's guess.

Twenty-two Indians and Mr. and Mrs. Thomas, the caretakers, comprised the population of Excursion Inlet. During World War II, 8000 troops had filled the barracks of this huge army depot. At a later date 60 American soldiers guarded the 700 German prisoners of war who had been transported to Excursion Inlet to demolish the unused barracks. The salvageable building materials were to be used to relieve the existing lumber shortage in Alaska. A few buildings and a vast network of roads were the only evidence left of this once-busy area.

Unable to entice anyone to explore with me, I put on my skis and took off alone through the three-foot fall of snow that blanketed the area. One road led into the woods past some of the buildings and was marked by signs in German. I could feel the loneliness those soldiers must have experienced in this wilderness. At another crossroads I imagined the bustle and clatter of the 8000 troops. It was a haunting place in which to wander alone.

Eventually I found a road that wound upward through the trees. The urge to see where it led drove me farther than I had planned. More and more sunlight and blue sky appeared until, at the top, I came to a large ice-covered reservoir and a viewpoint. Again, as I stood up there looking into the fog that covered everything below me, and out across the endless mountains, I had a peculiar feeling of being surrounded by the thoughts of all the unknown people who had been stationed there, either despising the remoteness or appreciating the beauty.

When I returned, the bustle of the ship and a delicious turkey dinner cooked by Dr. Krusich quickly brought me back to the present. After we stuffed ourselves and sat in the dining salon talking, listening to records and writing letters, the ghostly feelings I had felt so strongly a few hours before disappeared.

Monday we took care of the 24 residents and made the ship ready to leave early the next morning.

Juneau
Tuesday, February 18, to Tuesday, February 25

On our return to Juneau, we found an atmosphere totally different from any we had experienced on our previous stops. A bustling city replaced the small relaxed town. Restaurants and bars overflowed. Knots of people, talking excitedly, were everywhere. The health department offices bulged with doctors, nurses and sanitarians from all over the Territory. "The legislature is in session" explained everything. The excitement was contagious. The very future of the Alaska Department of Health's expanding new programs was at stake, dependent on decisions made in the next few days.

In addition to the overwhelming health problems, the legislators were under strong pressure to make other drastic changes. Statehood was on everyone's mind. Some violently opposed it, afraid of taxation, but most of the people we had met wanted control of their government and resources. They wanted to regulate and tax salmon canneries, to break the shipping monopoly and exorbitant freight rates, to get a fair share of federal highway funds, and to settle the aboriginal land claims. These topics had been discussed everywhere we had visited, and were expressed even more vehemently in Juneau. The Territory of Alaska appeared to be on the verge of a crisis due to the neglect of the U.S. Congress, which year after year had refused to act, or acted only for the benefit of powerful absentee interests.

It was a time for change. In 1946, Alaskans had voted in favor of statehood, and the hope was that maybe, just maybe, the Alaska Legislature might accomplish something for the good of Alaska. The Department of Health under Dr. Albrecht's able and aggressive direction was making good progress. In addition to the Alaska Legislature's large appropriation to fight tuberculosis, Dr. Albrecht had successfully prodded the United States Congress to approve significant and unusually generous funds as well as surplus equipment and facilities to help the territory's health program. Seventy years of neglect was ending at long last.

Visitors and friends from every part of Alaska swarmed over the *Hygiene*. Members of the legislature eagerly examined the result of their appropriations, and on the whole expressed approval. We were showered with invitations to dinners and parties.

One evening we met Dr. Elaine Schwinge, a jolly young medic, who showed us pictures of "her" truck unit. While they traveled Alaska's highways, they encountered all the problems of extreme cold and isolation encountered by the *Hygiene*. In addition, they had to find food and lodging with every move, do their own cooking, and cope with truck breakdowns. Dr. Schwinge's enthusiasm was contagious, and I wished we had her on the *Hygiene*.

Two additions to the *Hygiene* were to expand our physical and mental horizons. A 15-foot inboard motor launch replaced the old rowboat. It was driven like a car, and even had a reverse gear. We hoped it would provide transportation at villages with no docks, especially around Kodiak Island and in the Bering Sea. Although it was a far cry from the deep-sided dories of Kodiak Island, it was a vast improvement. I could hardly wait to learn how to run it. Larry did not trust me to take his new boat out by myself, but he allowed me to practice running and landing it if I had a crew member with me.

The second addition, we learned to our delight, was Dr. Elaine Schwinge, the 26-year-old physician of the highway unit. She had been assigned to help out on the *Hygiene* through February and into March, or until the highways became passable in the north. One year out of medical school, she was conscientious, energetic, and full of fun. We soon found out she loved to tell stories. One of the first she told us was how she happened to be where she was.

"While I was on the plane from Seattle to Juneau coming to this job, I asked myself, 'Why am I doing this?' I answered myself, 'There are several reasons.' One was that I had told my mother, who died while I was in school, that I wanted to be a missionary doctor, and she approved. Well, working for the territory wasn't exactly being a missionary, but the Eskimos did need medical help.

"Another more recent reason was that I had been working as an intern in a downtown Philadelphia hospital. It was noted as the worst hospital in Philadelphia—people shot each other, policemen beat up patients, and we were so short-staffed that I was working at least 80 to 90 hours a week, starting at 7:30 Thursday morning and getting off at noon or 7 p.m. Saturday. I was so exhausted that I would drop in bed completely clothed at times, only to be bothered by the telephone on emergencies throughout the time I was on call. With only a couple of days off between stints, this went on for a year. In fact, I was so exhausted at the end of it that I called my father after I had my medical license and internship completed. I said, 'Dear Dad, I appreciate the fact that you have paid for my medical education, but I have decided that I don't want to be a doctor.' So he said to me, 'OK, Elaine, you're such a nice person, whatever you want to be you can be. What would you like to be?' I said, 'I think I'll be a secretary because I can work from nine to five.' He said, 'Fine, I'll help you get to be a secretary.'

"But soon my conscience began to bother me and I thought, really, I have this medical degree; how in the world can I survive as a human being and still practice medicine? I looked in the Journal of the American Medical Association and there was an advertisement—'Wanted ship's doctor in Alaska.' I immediately looked up to see where Alaska was and found that it was nearly the size of the United States and that it only had a few thousand people in it. I said to myself, that's not more than two per square mile, I think that I can probably manage. Therefore I wrote and applied for the job, and to my amazement I got it, and here I am, hoping that I can survive."

After Dr. Schwinge joined us, mealtime discussions ranged over a wide variety of subjects—from the structure of the atom to world politics to Christianity. Everyone joined in, and mealtimes were fun, not just a time to gripe about conditions. The sea was not Dr. Schwinge's favorite place, but she did not dwell on that, except to tell Kitty and me she would much rather be on her truck unit, even if it was cold. At least it did not give her a queasy stomach.

I had been feeling a bit lonely the last few weeks because Kitty and Gus were spending more and more free time in long and serious conversations. As soon as Dr. Schwinge came aboard, I found a kindred spirit who shared my love of exploring.

After a week of frenetic activity in Juneau, we were eager to be underway again. Rex, the first mate, had left abruptly, delaying our departure for a day because the deckhand position was also unfilled. Art Berthold, an old seaman, replaced Rex, and Jim Brumbaugh filled the deckhand position. Then we headed for Kake, a village of about 300, located on the northwest end of Kupreanof Island.

Kake
Wednesday, February 26, to Wednesday, March 12

Approaching Kake, Larry cautiously followed the channel, noted for its rocks and reefs. Dr. Schwinge and I were in the pilot house peering through the fog at the numerous islands and rocks that lined the route. Suddenly we heard the distant sound of band music, and then lights shone dimly. Had the village turned out to welcome us? We saw no one. Larry continued on his course for a mile and a half, and we tied up at the cannery dock.

The watchman pointed out the trail to Kake. Dr. Schwinge, Kitty and I decided to walk over and let the village teachers and nurse know we had arrived. Slogging through snow and darkness, the mile and a half seemed like five. The lights of the village and a store with people in it looked mighty good. When they heard we had hiked from the cannery, one of the men asked, "Did you come without a gun?"

Kitty looked at me and I, reading her thoughts said, "Yes we did, aren't all the bears hibernating now?"

The man replied, "Not bears, wolves. It's been such a hard winter they have been coming into town and killing our dogs. They probably won't attack three people, so if you stay together you'll no doubt be safe."

With that piece of news snug in the back of our minds, we found the nurse, Mrs. Stansfield, and informed her the *Hygiene* was at the cannery dock, and we hoped to start work in the morning. She suggested that it would be much easier to transport the people to the boat if we could anchor in front of the village. The long walk would be hard for some of them. We understood and agreed to pass the message on to the captain. On our way back to the ship we practically glued ourselves together. We heard rustlings and padded footfalls behind every tree.

Larry found a good anchorage directly in front of the town next to a cluster of fishing boats. The new motor launch busily ferried us and our patients back and forth between shore and the *Hygiene* during the stay at Kake.

In this village of 350 people, the unpainted, two-story houses, most with electric lights, running water, and outdoor privies, impressed Dr. Schwinge. She commented that, on the whole, the community was more advanced than the interior villages she had served with the truck unit.

The number of people infected with TB, however, was frightening. Mrs. Stansfield, the local Alaska Native Service nurse, reported that eight deaths from tuberculosis had occurred since her arrival in June, nine months previously. She had sent eight other far-advanced cases to sanitariums. We found 62 suspicious cases including two children with bone tuberculosis.

Education, one of our most important tools, was not working in this village. The people did not show up for classes or movies. Kitty came up with the idea of having various organizations in town, such as the Salvation Army, the Presbyterian Church, and the village council sponsor evening meetings. The excellent Salvation Army band (which we had heard practicing on our arrival) played at some of them, and the Presbyterian Church choir sang at others. Then we showed our movies. The doctors, nurses, and village leaders all spoke, defin-

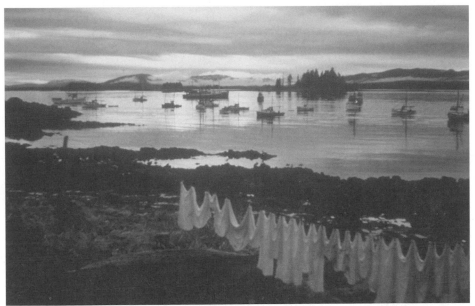

Kake

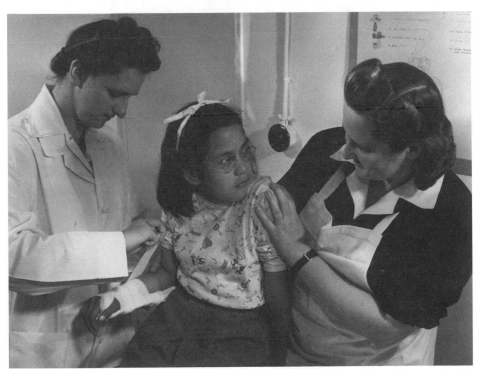

Dr. Schwinge, Kitty, and a patient

ing the problems and some of the solutions. This approach resulted in greatly improved attendance and enthusiasm. Dr. Krusich was pleased that all the patients with positive sputums attended her final meeting. Four of them were young people, and three had families with young children.

Kake was famous for its basketball team. Before a game, Dr. Krusich presented a class which was well attended and heeded. Earlier, during the physical examinations, she discovered that one team member who had been hospitalized for TB had left the hospital against the doctor's advice. The young man umpiring the game also had a positive X-ray and sputum. Several team members took the information seriously and refused to continue playing on the team. A few of the enthusiastic fans thought the *Hygiene* had done the town a disservice by weakening their championship team.

Between their own programs and the *Hygiene's* activities, the people of Kake had a busy schedule. Again the town included us in their social life. The Presbyterian and Salvation Army churches were active and met the needs of the people, who participated enthusiastically in the band and choir. Basketball was the main activity at that time of year, and it involved the entire town. Drinking was more of a problem than at Hoonah because the mail boat brought liquor in. This made some of the people quite indignant because they had voted to be a dry town.

The weather moderated while we were anchored at Kake, and the program moved forward smoothly. Wind and waves seemed to be in the past—until 4 a.m. one morning. A rhythmic banging on the hull, as if a giant were knocking to be let in, awakened us. Soon we heard Indian voices shouting, and pounding footsteps running back and forth on our deck. The howling wind had whipped up some good-sized waves. Then we heard the engines start, and the frantic sounds became somewhat calmer. Kitty called out as I passed her door, "What happened?"

"I don't know."

In our robes we went to the galley where we found the rest of the staff trying to figure out what had occurred. We were moving away from the village. We could see lights moving around our former anchorage. Then our anchor went down, and the bells rang to shut down the engines.

The story came out in bits and pieces as various crew members came in with their versions. A blast of wind had blown the *Hygiene* toward the *Helen G.* and the *Valhalla,* two small fishing boats anchored near her. The wind was so strong that we had dragged our anchor along the bottom until it fouled the anchor lines on the two fishing boats closest to us. The impact awakened a fisherman who was spending the night on his boat. He sounded an alarm that awakened our crew and the Natives ashore. Art and Jim pulled up our anchor and untangled it from the other boats' anchor lines.

While they were doing that, the wind swung the *Hygiene* so her propeller became entangled in another anchor line. Total darkness added to the confusion. Gus could not start the engine to move out until the men freed the propeller. Meanwhile, the wind was blowing our big ship closer and closer to the anchored fishing fleet. Finally Art gave the all clear on the propeller, and Gus immediately started the engines. Larry moved a safe distance away from the fishing fleet and anchored—over a reef, the Natives informed him the next day. Amazingly, daylight revealed no damage to any of the boats except for one lost anchor.

Lack of contact with the outside world was one unpleasant feature of shipboard life. Those of us on the medical staff especially longed for good music, news of the U.S., entertainment, and letters. We felt terribly isolated. At the store I noticed a short-wave radio for sale. After checking with Larry, I found it had the features I needed to operate on board—a good antenna and it used direct current. What joy to listen to a symphony! Sunday evenings my shipmates crowded into my little stateroom to listen to Edgar Bergen and Charlie McCarthy, a touch of home from that other world. Broadcasts from Hawaii and even Australia were especially exciting.

After we had worked in Kake for 10 days, it became apparent that two weeks was adequate to care for its problems. The services of two doctors and two nurses moved our program right along. Needless to say, I was very busy keeping up with them. Kitty and Dr. Schwinge helped me when they could.

On the last Sunday Dr. Schwinge and I cooked a turkey dinner. Neither one of us knew how to cook, and neither one of us had ever tried a turkey before. We were delighted when it turned out to be edible, no doubt due to the advice given to us by all the worried cooks who were going to have to eat it.

After that meal we went to a tea given by the Crutchers, teachers who had spent many years with the Eskimos in the Arctic. Their tales and obvious love of the Eskimo people raised our expectations of the *Hygiene's* trip north the following summer even more. They also told us stories about Kake's background. The town was in the throes of change. Only 80 years had passed since the last time Kake medicine men had led their war canoes south to raid and lay waste to Hydaburg. Reportedly the raiders carried off the Haida women and kept them prisoners for over a year. They made slaves of these prisoners, who had to do all the menial work for their captors. The villagers still looked on any domestic employment as beneath them. Many of the village elders found fault with the younger generation because they did not speak the Native tongue, eat Native foods, or follow their tribal customs.

Though they enthusiastically participated in the Presbyterian and Salvation Army churches, the townspeople would not allow anyone to kill the ravens that swarmed over the town. Their legends said that traditionally Raven had stolen light and given it to the world.

Even though isolated, the people living in their own villages seemed to be better off than those living in the larger cities, where they were treated as a lower class. In the villages, the Indians managed their own community affairs, and those who had the advantage of going away to school were most capable leaders. Alaska, as a whole, had come to a major crossroads. The legislature and the local people demonstrated this. Change was every-where—in culture, in customs, and in control.

Warm Springs Bay
Thursday, March 13, to Saturday, March 15

Angoon, on the west side of Admiralty Island, had no dock, so we made a water stop at the resort town of Warm Springs Bay. Its year-round population of 15 enjoyed the hot baths and acted as informal caretakers. The setting was breathtaking, a small quiet bay into which a beautiful large waterfall plunged. Tall green spruce trees covered with heavy snow formed the background. The houses, many uninhabited in winter, had "hot baths" running through them. The public baths were wooden tubs so slimy that it took a fair amount of courage to get into one.

Dr. Krusich decided to spend an extra day at the hot springs, even though two days earlier she had urged us to move the program along. Fog lengthened our stay to two days, and we only saw Dr. Krusich at meals. She seemed with-drawn and silent. Dr. Schwinge was by now getting an eyeful of Dr. Krusich's erratic behavior. Both Kitty and I hoped she would verify our reports of Krusich's unpredictable actions. It was important that the leadership of the doctor be as fine as possible—it not only affected the medical staff, but all the ship's person-nel and the entire program.

Angoon
Sunday, March 16, to Friday, March 21

Angoon, the first stop on our trial run the previous year, gave a choice of two anchorages. This time Larry decided, because of fickle weather, to anchor on the protected side of the point in spite of the extreme tidal currents which flowed through a narrow pass into a series of large bays. The tide formed fierce rips as it ran through this cleft. These did not bother the *Hygiene* at anchor, but at times they formed tidal bores or overfalls, with a one-to two-foot wall of water piling up on itself, or any small boat, as it reached the constricted pass. This anchorage provided plenty of excitement for us as we went back and forth in the launch.

One night Gus was bringing Kitty, Dr. Schwinge, and me back to the ship after a meeting. No one was thinking much about the tide. When we reached the narrowest part of the channel, the bow of the launch suddenly dived down and the sound of roaring water filled the air. The stern swung around, the propeller spinning in the air. The boat spun around again and water rushed over the stern. We hung on for dear life, and our eyes clung to the lights of the *Hygiene* as we turned and pitched. No one said anything for a few seconds after we came back to an even keel.

Then Gus's voice, cool as ever, said, "That was a big bore." Kitty laughed shakily, "Oh no, Gus, not a pun now. Will it happen again?"

"No," Gus replied as he revved up the motor. "We'll probably hit some good swirls and waves, but if the motor keeps going, we'll be OK."

Our work program and social life were similar to the routines in Kake, although Angoon's major problems were venereal disease and rheumatic fever. The X-ray survey revealed that the TB rate was much lower than in Kake and Hoonah. Here we saw the importance of the many records we kept. An Alaska Native Service nurse had been stationed here after our first visit, but for some unknown reason, she had none of the records. Thus one patient with a positive sputum, instead of going to a hospital, had a large wedding. Her husband knew nothing of her disease. He probably would not have married her if he had, because he already had several small children. Hospitalization for this young woman was imperative—and it was essential that the Native Service nurses had access to the records of the work being done on the Hygiene. Dr. Krusich planned to keep in touch to see that the young woman was indeed hospitalized.

We needed to improve this aspect of our program. Communication between the Territorial Department of Health and the Alaska Native Service did not appear efficient to those of us who, in a sense, were working for both of them. Even less communication had occurred between the two agencies before we started our program. Kitty, who had always considered herself a Territorial Department of Health nurse, was developing an intense sympathy and respect for the Alaska Native Service nurses. She did a great job in making the local nurses realize that they were an important part of the *Hygiene's* program.

Juneau
Saturday, March 22, to Friday, March 28

After we completed the work at Angoon and returned to Juneau, only Gus, Art, John, Kitty, and I stayed on. Dr. Krusich was leaving in May, only six weeks away, a day both Kitty and I had been anticipating. Dr. Schwinge, as planned, was rejoining her beloved highway unit. Larry had decided fishing was a better career than shepherding a temperamental doctor around, and he needed time to get his boat ready for the coming season.

Kitty and I were looking forward to the trip to the Bering Sea, but speculated on the character of our new shipmates. It was hard to adapt to the constantly changing crews. In spite of all the *Hygiene's* amenities, the long and irregular hours of work affected everyone on board, and crew members objected to the proportion of time spent away from major ports and their entertainments. We hoped the new doctor and captain would be an improvement.

Kitty wrote in her monthly nursing report, "Despite my philosophy of *trying* to remain removed from the crew and ship maintenance difficulties, it is hard to be unaffected by the frequent changes and disturbances in crew morale." I am sure her feelings for Gus made it even harder.

During the next week the replacement crew and a secretary were hired. It took a few days to get the men sorted out. The new Skipper, Lynn Crosby, was a chubby, talkative man whose experience was with small boats. Mr. Brown, pushing 60, replaced Jessie. A tall, kindly man from Texas, his paunch hung over his belt to an amazing degree. He served great quantities of excellent food, never grumbled, and believed a good meal or snack would take care of any problem.

The legislature was still in session, and Kitty and I had some time to listen in again. We were happy to hear that the Department of Health appropriations had passed earlier. At this stage, the legislators were tired. Anger and frustration were rampant. When Kitty contrasted it to the U.S. Congress she had seen in Washington, D.C., where half the members were absent, asleep, or reading their papers during debate, the Alaskans' dedication impressed her. All the

Alaskan legislators were present, and their intensity was exhilarating. March 27 was the last day for them to meet, but at 11:30 p.m. they were still arguing, so they stopped the clock and continued all night and into the next day before they wound up the session.

The main topic of conversation in Juneau during this stopover was the first live symphony orchestra ever to perform there. The concert was to be on March 26 at the Twentieth Century Theater. Everyone we knew was going, and when Kitty and I learned we would be in town, we found, with some difficulty, three tickets and invited Dr. Schwinge to join us.

Our lives had not been completely without music. We had enjoyed the various dance bands in the villages. We had my radio and a record player with a few classical records on board ship, but the crew objected to "long-hair" music, as they called it. We had almost forgotten how satisfying and uplifting a good symphony concert could be.

It is doubtful if any orchestra ever received a more enthusiastic ovation than was given by this audience. As we floated out the theater door, the last strains of the music still in our heads, waving curtains of filmy colored lights filled the sky. It was as though the heavens had heard and were drawing their many layers of colored curtains back and forth. This tremendous display of northern lights impressed even the old-time Alaskans.

Ketchikan
Sunday, March 30, to Monday, March 31

On Friday, March 28, we left Juneau with a full crew and medical staff. We arrived in Ketchikan on Seward's Day weekend, an Alaskan holiday honoring the United States purchase of the territory from the Russians. For a change, the weather was beautiful. Some of the friends we had made during the survey in July came to greet us. Dixie, Ketchikan's bacteriologist, and John, a friend of hers, invited me to go fishing with them and John caught a nice halibut—cause for a party.

Kitty had been immediately whisked off by Rudd, a young man who had become interested in her during the survey. After Dixie phoned around and found them, we gathered to feast on the fish and catch up with what had been happening in each other's lives.

Southeastern Alaskans had a great interest in the remote sections of their territory. They heard stories from fishermen, officials who made surveys, and politicians, but no ferries or tour boats yet existed, so the average citizen could not travel to see the country. Kitty showed slides of our trip and gave our friends a better idea of what lay to the north of them.

Ketchikan was a lively town, and the people were active on many fronts. The hottest issue at that time was whether or not to chlorinate the local water supply. A large and vocal group believed they had the best and purest water in the world, and they did not want anyone poisoning it. Dixie and other members of the health department were concerned, because every summer an outbreak of gastroenteritis occurred. After they had checked every conceivable cause for this disease, water was the only suspect left. The water supply came from a protected lake high above the town. Dixie agreed that campers or hikers could not contaminate it, but she knew that somehow, somewhere in the system, the water was being polluted, and she would have to clearly prove it to the opposition.

One day the sanitarian looked out his window at the bay in front of the town, as he pondered the problem. Idly, he watched the activities of the many seagulls on the waterfront. Gulls were on every piling and lined up on the roofs of cannery and dock sheds above the water. Whenever someone on a boat threw garbage over the side, a swarm of seagulls wheeled about and then settled in the water to feed. Suddenly the picture was clear.

Ketchikan, as did other towns, poured its untreated sewage into the salt water in the bay, where it was eventually carried off by the tide. As the garbage and fish waste from the canneries floated back and forth on the sewage-laden water, large numbers of seagulls busily ate it. Then, mused the sanitarian, what did they do? He watched and sure enough great numbers of them flew up to Ketchikan's "clean and pure" water supply, where they paddled around and washed the sewage from their feathers and feet.

Members of the health department then isolated the organism causing the gastroenteritis from a patient, the seagull's feet, and the lake water. Ketchikan's water supply, after many more verbal battles, was chlorinated, and the yearly epidemic of waterborne disease ended. The moral was, as Dixie said, "It does pay to look out the window."

Metlakatla
Tuesday, April 1, to Saturday, April 12

We were hard at work in Metlakatla after the lovely weekend in Ketchikan, where we had been able to get away from the ship and talk to different people. Kitty had enjoyed the attention Rudd paid to her. Gus, however, was intensely jealous because Kitty had spent an evening with Rudd. He accused her of having a boyfriend in every port and was grumpy with all of us. At that point Kitty decided never to settle down to one man, unless she was married. Marriage must have been somewhat on her mind, since she was embroidering a linen tablecloth and collecting china cups and saucers. At this particular time the romance of Kitty and Gus looked rather hopeless.

Since our last visit, the town council of Metlakatla had found an excellent nurse, Mrs. Miller, and a lay nurse, Priscilla. They had neatly filed records of the positive TB cases from the year before. After identifying suspected cases of venereal disease, they had insisted that these people see the doctors in Ketchikan.

Even with this improved health care, we were puzzled by the residents' definite lack of interest in our program. At first we attributed this to the proximity of Ketchikan's doctors, nurses, and hospital, but as the week wore on, we felt a sense of excitement pervading the village. More and more of the visits to the ship for X-rays and consultations were either canceled or forgotten. Groups of housewives gathered in serious conversations over fences and on porches. Knots of men constantly formed on the docks and streets.

On our arrival, the mayor had invited us to a reception the following week. This often happened in the small towns, and we had not thought much about it. We were aware that a property lease was being renegotiated, but not until we saw many "city-type" men in business suits with briefcases did we realize the importance of the occasion. The federal government through the Civil Aeronautics Authority had leased a flat peninsula on the southwest end of Annette Island, which was owned by the Metlakatlans. The lease was about to terminate. The CAA and the town of Ketchikan depended on this rare piece of flat land for their airfield and wanted to renew the lease.

The night of the reception, a group of us went to the town hall, where the village officials greeted us warmly and introduced us to our hostess, who remained with us through the evening. She explained that the reception was for government officials from the different departments, who were in town to negotiate the lease contracts. She then led us to our table and described the program for the evening. We appreciated her graciousness because this was a supper for about 200 people, and we would have felt lost in the crowd.

Beautifully set tables decorated with daffodils and Easter lilies filled the large room. Each table had a hostess and several helpers who took care of the people sitting there. They served a delicious meal of cold meats, salads, rolls, relishes, ice cream, and cookies, with tea and coffee.

The apparent ease and speed with which they served such a large group was impressive and showed a high degree of organization and cooperation. Each woman was responsible for one table. She used her own linens, silver and china, and then took them off in a basket to be washed later at home. The hostesses then could join in the dancing and enjoy the fun after dinner. A 20-piece band and three singers provided entertainment during dinner. A Metlakatlan master of ceremonies made the introductions with humor and great poise. The mayor gave a short speech. Both men were totally at ease and most articulate. After the banquet and speeches, the dancing began. I thought if the men were as good at negotiating as their wives were at entertaining, they could not lose. The negotiations apparently reached a successful conclusion, because the Army and Ketchikan continued using the airfield.

The *Hygiene* had been described in many ways at various times and locations. Some had seen her anchored in a pleasant bay when we had a Sunday off and called her a pleasure yacht. Others, seeing crew members and even the doctor drunk when they were ashore, labeled it as a group of people on a drunken spree. Kitty and I were upset at being associated with this reputation. That evening when Metlakatla's mayor, John Smith, relayed a message to us from a Pan American Airway pilot, we were overjoyed that some of the gossip about us was good. The message: "The *Hygiene* was the nearest thing anyone would see to Christ walking on the waters."

Ketchikan to Juneau
Monday, April 14, to Saturday, April 19

We stopped off in Ketchikan to swing the compass and then spent the night in Wrangell on our way north. I found a small totem pole that had been made into a lamp and a paddle carved with the raven design for my kayak. Our time in Juneau was filled with ordering supplies for the long summer trip. Again we would be months away from any source of supplies.

Haines and Klukwan
Sunday, April 20, to Monday, April 28

After our brief stop in Juneau, we proceeded to Haines. The area included three communities, their total population about 500. The dock at Haines proper was too small for a ship the size of the *Hygiene*, so we tied up a mile south at Chilkoot Barracks.

Formerly known as Fort Seward, this settlement had been the only Army post in Alaska until the war. A group of veterans had recently formed a cooperative community there. Living in well-built two- and three-story houses situated around a parade ground, the members had all the modern conveniences, including a large, sturdy dock left from the Army days. All they needed were ingenuity and hard work to start some lucrative projects. The members had to support themselves and pay off certain lawsuits that had been incurred in the purchase of the facility. Enthusiasm ran high, no doubt helped by a small cannery, a sawmill, and an abundance of good land for homesteading. An added bonus, this area enjoyed some of the best weather in Southeast Alaska.

Haines proper was a mixed white and Indian village. These peaceful, friendly Natives were descended from the smart and aggressive Chilkat tribesmen who, in the early days, were middlemen between the fur hunters in the interior and the coastal fur traders.

The totally Indian village of Klukwan was 22 miles up the river over a very bad road. The road, such as it was, continued into Canada to join the Alaska Highway. The people of Klukwan, excellent craftsmen, noted for their rare Chilkat blankets woven from mountain goat hair, were suspicious of outsiders, and for good reason. The early missionaries had destroyed most of their carvings, masks, and blankets because they were ignorant of their significance. Fortunately the tribe had been able to save a few pieces by hiding them, and had secretly created others. They trusted and honored us by inviting us to a Native dance in which they used beautiful specimens of their famous blankets and awesome masks. One young fellow sold us intricately carved silver bracelets, pins, and earrings made from silver dollars.

Haines boasted both a Native and a Territorial school. The two principals and the Presbyterian minister gave taxi service between the communities for the X-ray survey. Our work concentrated on examining the schoolchildren and the routine X-ray program. No positive films showed up in Haines, but three turned up in Klukwan, a more primitive town.

One Sunday afternoon Jim, the deckhand, and Morris, our redheaded mess boy, and I took the new launch to a mink farm about two miles across the bay to see if anyone there needed an X-ray. The trip over was most pleasant, and the fellows let me run the boat. The mink rancher came down to the dock to greet us, wondering where we had come from. Jim, in his best public relations manner said, "We're from the *Hygiene*, the public health ship over at Chilkoot Dock for a couple of weeks. Come on over and get your X-ray. This is Susie, she takes them." I seconded the invitation and asked if we could see the mink.

"Sure, come on up. It's too bad you couldn't come next weekend," the farmer explained. "We have 350 mink. The females are all pregnant and their pups are due in about two more days."

I admired the different colors of the furry little creatures. Some were white, some red, and the most beautiful were a silvery blue. "These," he explained as he held a silvery blue mother-to-be, "are mutations and cost $500 apiece."

Entranced with this "ranch," I was all set to learn more until Jim pointed to the wind in the treetops and suggested it might be wise to head back before a full-fledged storm struck. The farmer agreed and promised to try and get over for his X-ray.

The water was somewhat rough as we left. I had great confidence in the launch until, as the wind constantly increased, a short, high chop built up. One of the boat's faults then became apparent. It threw up tremendous amounts of spray, so much that some of the time I felt I was under water. Jim was most encouraging and let me do all the navigating, although he did point out land-marks, as I was having trouble seeing through all the water on my glasses. He constantly reassured me that everything was all right, we were just wet. I was glad I had an old "sea dog" along. We were soaked to the skin by the time I made the landing at the *Hygiene*. After a change into dry clothes and a gallon of hot clam chowder, we were warm again and happy with our adventure. I was perfectly content to sit and knit and listen to my radio that night.

As I knitted I could not help thinking about Jim. His smashed nose, scarred cheek and missing upper teeth gave a clue to his past life. If he had worn a cutlass and walked on a peg-leg he would have formed a perfect picture of a pirate. Gentle brown eyes contradicted the rest of the appearance of this 42-year-old man. The tattoos on his muscular arms gave a clue to his interests—each exhibited a large picture of a beautiful woman. Surrounding these major works of art, many small cherubs and anchors entwined around each other, to give an idea of Jim's views on family life.

Jim had only a third-grade education, but he was reading the Bible for the third time, claiming it meant more to him each time. He could quote Robert Service at great length, and Shakespeare was one of his favorite authors. He read and thought about almost any subject of general interest, and expressed his opinions more colorfully than those on board who were supposed to be educated. In spite of his tough appearance and stories of drunken brawls and fights that sent him either to the hospital or jail—where he had apparently spent a lot of time—Jim was a gentle and kindly man. I realized that this apparent roughneck, who had at first somewhat intimidated me, now was a friend whom I respected and enjoyed.

Skagway
Monday, April 28, to Saturday, May 3

A short run to the end of Lynn Canal brought us to the long dock at Skagway. Steep cliffs rose sheer out of the water, and the dock rose parallel to them. Ships' names painted in many hues covered the rocky wall to an unbelievable height. We speculated how the painters gained such altitudes.

Kitty and I found that our bikes were the most practical way of traversing the long dock and the short road to town. We had no trouble getting there because the wind helped. It blew down the bay toward the town all the time, day and night. But once, on a return trip, it blew so hard it brought us to a standstill on a perfectly level road. The Indian name for Skagway means "Home of the North Wind."

While Haines was thought to be the "coming" town in Alaska, if the highway was kept open, Skagway was still reliving its past of the '98 gold rush days. The people in this mainly white town made their money working for the railroad and catering to tourists. A kangaroo court fined all the males who did not grow summer beards.

The city owned and maintained most of the town's historic buildings. Whenever a tour boat tied up at the dock, men with beards and women in flowing skirts greeted it and proceeded to re-enact the shooting of Soapy Smith, one of the town's notorious characters. Work prevented us from watching these organized presentations. We had to be content with hearing and reading about the hardships of the gold rush days, Chilkoot Pass, and the building of the White Pass and Yukon railroad.

One of our patients told us about Mrs. Pullen, a young widow with four small children. She had arrived in Skagway in 1897 with $7. By baking apple pies, she made enough money to buy some horses. With them she earned more money by carrying freight to the bottom of the Chilkoot and White Pass trails. She finally ended up with enough money to build a hotel, the Pullen House. Except for the fact that now only 400 to 500 people lived in the town instead of ten to twenty thousand, we found it hard to believe the date was May 1947 and not 1898, as we wandered around with the costumed citizens.

One evening Kitty and I stopped at the old Pullen House, part of which was a museum. The door was open, so we walked in. Looking around the dimly lit lobby, we felt like intruders, since no one was there. Seeing a lighted doorway at the end of a long dark hall, we started toward it. As we approached, a ghostly, pale old lady with white hair piled on top of her head came into view. Dressed in a long white nightshirt, she was sitting at a table drinking coffee.

When we drew near, her hand fluttered, and we could not tell whether she meant for us to come in or go away—so we went in. Apparently it was the right decision.

She started talking in a quavery voice, "I'm Mrs. Pullen, please come in and make yourselves comfortable."

Kitty and I introduced ourselves and Kitty asked, "Is there a museum here?"

"Eh, What's that, young lady? You'll have to speak up, I'm a little hard of hearing. My daughter will be right back, We will have a room for you very soon. I'm 87 years old, you know. Not as spry as I used to be. Come, let me show you the museum."

Mrs. Pullen stood up and tottered down the hall to some display cases containing Soapy Smith's guns and brass knuckles. At that point her daughter arrived and took her mother back to her room, explaining, "Mother is quite deaf and sometimes her mind wanders. Please make yourselves at home." She turned on some lights so we could appreciate the historic hotel more fully. We had trouble deciding where the museum stopped and the hotel began.

The many bars and the atmosphere of the town got to several of the crew. At first, only a couple of crew members went up town and came back aboard drunk. On another night several more came back and had a fight with the captain, whom they did not respect. He was quite opinionated and very stubborn. Gus thought he lacked experience on boats the size of the *Hygiene*. On our last night the doctor and most of the crew had gone up to town and were roaring drunk when Kitty and I returned from a pleasant dinner and evening with the minister and his family. The wild party on the *Hygiene* was reverberating against the cliffs. Quietly we slipped into our staterooms, turned out the lights, locked the doors, and pretended we were not there.

I lay in my bunk listening to the senseless cursing and fighting that spilled out onto the deck every now and then, wondering what it was that made people lose interest in the exciting and beautiful world around them—a world filled with friendly, interesting people. What caused them to go to bars with the same group they were apparently bored and unhappy with, to sit around and hash over the same old gripes, while drinking themselves into a stupor? It all seemed so pointless. It was a shame to see that the major problems of Alaska regarding alcoholism were also prevalent among many of the *Hygiene's* personnel.

The next day the doctor, the captain, and all the crew—except Gus, Kitty, and me had packed their bags, planning to leave the ship when it returned to Juneau. I told Kitty, "I've enjoyed most of these people as individuals, but I'm glad we're going to have a fresh start for our second year afloat." Kitty agreed.

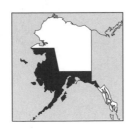

5
The
Bering Sea

The most difficult waters of all were in the Bering Sea, which freezes from
sometime in September until sometime in May. Travel in the northern sec-
tions is limited to about three months. Many parts of the area are shallow,
even miles out from shore. The demarcation between land and sea is vague,
with the sea bottom rising to within a few feet of its surface. The shore is
covered with deltas, swamps, and tundra for many miles inland. Add fog
and strong winds—the result is an area not often visited by outsiders. The
people living there were for the most part Eskimos who did not speak En-
glish and had a traditional lifestyle.

Juneau: Preliminaries
Sunday, May 4, to Sunday, June 8

THE LONG-AWAITED ASSIGNMENT to work in the villages around the
Bering Sea came in May. We had a month to prepare for a six-month journey
to the north. Conferences and lists filled our days. The *Hygiene* went to dry dock for
repairs on her keel and rudder. Two more water tanks were also added below the
clinic deck. We had heard that the Bering Sea would present a major problem in
procuring fresh water. The new tanks were supposed to be the answer. Dr. Schwinge,
to Kitty's and my delight, was to be the physician on board until some time in July.

While the ship was in dry dock, I flew to Seattle for dental work. Shortly after
I arrived, my mother had a heart attack and was rushed to the hospital. Her first
concern was that I continue on my trip north. Excited by my adventures, she
was determined that her frail body was not going to spoil them. When her

condition stabilized rapidly, the doctor agreed with her. He calmed my concerns by frankly discussing them.

"If you stay home, she could just as well have another attack while you are at the grocery store. You can't stop living and wait for it."

The decision on whether to go or stay was a hard one. I knew how inaccessible I would be if my mother had further troubles. On the other hand, there was no time to train a replacement for me. The window of weather during which we could work in the Bering Sea was so short that every day was important. Nor did I want to miss the trip north.

At my mother's urging, I found a reliable friend to stay with her and take over her care. I left Seattle with a worried mind, but I was determined to write such good letters that Mother could vicariously enjoy my experiences in the Bering Sea.

Just before I left Seattle, I received a wire from the Juneau office authorizing me to purchase a much-needed binocular microscope to replace the old monocular scope I had been struggling with. This would make the lab work much more comfortable, but I had to get the heavy microscope to Juneau before the ship left in three days. That meant I had to carry it onto the plane as hand baggage. (In those days all baggage was carefully weighed and recorded.) I walked to the plane with the heavy scope in its case, trying to look as though it weighed no more than a purse.

I was about to heave a sigh of relief when a pleasant male voice from behind me said, "Here, let me give you a hand with that."

Looking up, I mumbled something like, "It's really not very heavy," as I saw the bars on the captain's shoulders. "Oh, oh," I thought, "he probably won't let me keep it."

"There you are," he said as he handed the heavy case to the stewardess, with no mention of excess weight.

The Hygiene gleamed with a new coat of paint, and a formidable stack of boxed supplies filled the X-ray and laboratory sections. I had only two days to check them against my lists and stow each item safely for traveling. Every available space, including some new cupboards, was jammed full by the time I emptied the last box.

Juneau to Sitka
Sunday, June 8, to Tuesday, June 10

At 6 a.m. on June 8, 1947, the *Hygiene's* engines roared to life. A sparkling Sunday morning initiated this voyage of a lifetime. We were eager and happy to be on our way to Sitka, our first destination. There, awaiting us, was a dental X-ray machine, the last piece of equipment to be installed in the *Hygiene's* new dental clinic. A tiny space for the dental chair and equipment had been built into one corner of the waiting room during the past month. The dentist and his assistant, whom he had married recently, would join us in the Bering Sea coastal area.

Our new captain, George Kippola from Tacoma, had been master of the Alaska Department of Transport Services vessels and was well qualified for the job on the *Hygiene*. Shortly after breakfast he called all of the ship's personnel together and gave instructions for fire and lifeboat drill. That was the first time anyone had done that on the *Hygiene*. He also discussed his policy on drinking. No liquor would be allowed on board, either underway or in port. The crew grumbled that the captain was getting carried away with his own importance. We on the medical staff thought he was very wise.

Jessie, who had taken a two-month break, returned to cook, much to our delight. Del had been promoted to bosun's mate. Newlyweds Sigurd Harris, secretary, and Red Harris, assistant engineer, had just joined us. John Bergquist, an old sea dog, was first mate, and Wayne LaCassa, a cocky young fellow, was the new deckhand. The mess boy was Ronald Heilman, an irrepressible, rotund man in his forties. He had worked for years at a routine job in an auto factory in Detroit, all the while reading and dreaming about Alaska. Ronald was a delight from the start. Nothing ruffled him, and he was so filled with enthusiasm and book lore about Alaska that it was a joy to be around him. Excited about everything, he could hardly believe he had actually escaped from the dull life and job in which he had been trapped for so many years.

After lunch we turned west into Peril Strait, very suitably named. Sections of the narrow channel seemed barely wide enough for us to pass through. The powerful tide rips swung our 114-foot ship about in a frightening manner. But the beautiful scenery soon entranced us. Snowcapped mountains rose on the port side. Some were needle-pointed peaks; others had hanging glaciers glistening in the sunlight. Eagles perched on their nests on both sides of the narrow channel. Deer skittered off the beaches as we passed. Whales cavorted around us, their foamy white exhalations showing clearly against the dark background of trees. A strong, fishy odor assailed our senses as we passed them.

Sitka to Seward
Wednesday, June 11, to Friday, June 13

It was 10 p.m. when we tied up at the Standard Oil dock in Sitka. We took off to see the sights of the historic town, since it was still light. Gus and Kitty lagged behind the rest of us, walking hand in hand, deep in conversation. Circled by snowcapped mountains and many jewel-like islands, the well-kept community enchanted us.

The first thing Monday morning, Dr. Schwinge called Mr. Andreason, the Alaska Native Service (ANS) administrator, to locate the dental X-ray unit. He advised her that we should move to the ANS dock on Japonsky Island across the channel from Sitka. The dock was closer to the needed equipment, and it would save the $35 per night docking fee at the Standard Oil dock. We moved over immediately.

Mr. Andreason also recommended that one of the town's experienced electricians put the dental X-ray unit together. Dr. Schwinge had been under the impression that Gus could just plug it in, but she found it consisted of four parts and was a complicated wiring job. As time was precious, she thought that it best be done quickly, so she hired the electrician to work with Gus.

This would enable Dr. Marshall, a TB consultant, who was hitching a ride with us, to reach Seward sooner. From there he was scheduled to start case-finding with his portable X-ray unit. He would travel by plane throughout the northern areas not covered by the mobile health truck or the *Hygiene*.

While Gus and the electrician worked on the installation, Dr. Schwinge and I went to the TB sanitarium on Alice Island. The complex had been part of a large Navy base during the war. The Territorial Department of Health and the Bureau of Indian Affairs were converting it into a sanitarium, an orthopedic hospital, and a vocational school. This large acquisition had been the hope and talk of the health department for nearly a year.

One of the Catholic sisters took us through the facility. At that time it had the capacity to care for about 250 patients, with the ability to expand if Congress appropriated the funds. Money was available for only one electrician to care for two large hospitals and one 500-student school. When we found that the electrician was paid $16.50 for five hours' work, we wondered why the government could not come up with the money to run the place adequately. We decided so much money was going to war-torn Europe that none was left for the neglected native-born citizens of the territory who definitely needed help, maybe more than the victims of the war.

In spite of the lack of personnel, the tour left us with the impression of a light and airy atmosphere in a place of hope and good cheer. We were excited to share the enthusiasm of the people working there and to see the development of so many desperately needed facilities.

In medical matters, ingenuity was the name of the game. In the children's wing, the nurses were still struggling with basic equipment built for adults.

For example, when they needed ankle cuffs for the orthopedic cases, they went to the surplus property supplies and salvaged parts of suspenders, tourniquets, and the leather tongues in shoes. In spite of these difficulties, the nurses appeared to enjoy the challenge of improvising to meet the needs of child patients. Fifty boys and girls were there waiting for surgery and miscellaneous treatments; 300 more were on the list to be called.

That evening we gave the staff members from the TB sanitarium and the orthopedic hospital a tour of our facilities. Dr. Moore, the surgeon in charge, was away but Dr. Stein, a tall brunette with graying hair, stood in for him. A German-Jewish refugee, she had a terrific accent.

She told us of their troubles while opening the hospital. Supplies and clothing for the patients were nonexistent when she arrived. In fact, she had to set up the bed for the first patient. She kept harping continually to Dr. Rufus that she needed pajamas for her children.

"Finally," she laughed, "he fly from Juneau to Sitka with two suitcases. At the airport, in front of many of the men at the base, he proclaims, 'Dr. Stein, I brought your pajamas!'"

Rows of beds of confined children without toys, books, or even combs or toothbrushes made a pitiful sight in this modern shell of a hospital. But it was enlightening to see the efforts other people were making to help the children that we on the *Hygiene* were discovering and referring for care.

Just before the *Hygiene* was to leave at 10 a.m., Dr. Schwinge, Kitty, and I had a flying look at the building site of Baranof's castle. He had developed Sitka into the center of trading and culture on the Pacific coast. At one time while under Russian control it was called the Paris of the Pacific. His castle was gone, but the old Russian Orthodox church was still there on the main street. (It has since burned and been rebuilt from the original plans.)

While we crossed the Gulf all but four of the 14 aboard became seasick. As Dr. Schwinge put it, "It was unpleasant to have to lie down day and night and munch dry crackers and wonder if you dare empty out the pail now, or whether you'd just better stay down until the darn boat stayed upright." The two young deckhands who had tried to act like old sailors were also sick and most embarrassed. Down in the engine room, Gus pumped the bilges continuously. The ship had dried out while it was in dry dock, and an uncomfortable quantity of water was coming through the seams.

When we docked in Seward at 8 a.m., Captain Kippola and Dr. Schwinge decided to give the seasick crew one more day of rest, so they declared that Friday was Sunday. What a change from the year before! Dr. Marshall moved his X-ray equipment to the railroad express office and went on his way north. Dr. Schwinge asked Miss Arave, Seward's public health nurse, to take us out to the Seward sanitarium, Home in the Woods, to meet the Valles. Dr. Valle, an Argentinean by birth, was the only thoracic surgeon in the territory. He and his attractive wife took us on a tour of the sanitarium, explaining their troubles—patients running away, nurses leaving because of boredom, and meddling by the Methodist Church. Their good-natured way of putting up with "do withouts" spurred us to write to our own hospitals stateside for instruments and an anesthetist for them.

Seward to Dutch Harbor
Friday, June 13, to Tuesday, June 17

We left Seward for Dutch Harbor on calm seas under overcast skies. All except Sig, the new secretary, had gained their sea legs. She was still sick even though the water in the lee of Kodiak Island was dead calm.

On Monday morning, Dr. Schwinge did not show up after the second breakfast bell. She explained later she had heard both bells, but because the ship was rolling, she thought that it must be cloudy and rainy, and a good morning to sleep. Ronald, the mess boy and an avid photographer, as was the doctor, was concerned because we were passing a huge volcano. He knocked on her door again and called, until grumbling, she got up. Once up, she appreciatively shot many exposures of Mt. Pavlov, an active volcano, towering 8900 feet over the Alaska Peninsula. It had showered the country with ash in 1937.

False Pass marked the end of the mainland. Unimak Island crowned with Mt. Shishaldin (9387 ft.) began the Aleutian Chain. The mountain, sometimes called Smoking Moses, formed an almost perfect cone rising straight out of the sea. From Unimak Pass the Aleutians stretched westward beyond our route some 1300 miles toward Russian Kamchatka.

History began for Alaska in those treeless islands of volcanic origin. Bathed in a moist climate and covered with luxuriant growth of grasses and soft mosses, they endure winds so strong the insects cannot have wings because they will be blown into the sea.

Following Bering's third voyage, and before the Russian fur hunters arrived, the islands were inhabited by 25,000 peace-loving Aleuts. After being subjected to white men's diseases, these Natives suffered not only illnes and death, but slavery and senseless killing by the Russians' *promyshleniki*. The population at the time of our visit was scarcely 3000.

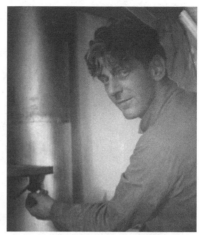

Right, top to bottom:
Gus, Wayne, Wendell.
Left: above, Captain Kippola;
below, Ronald with wakeup bell.

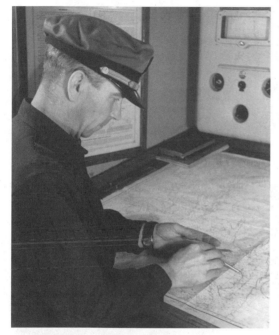

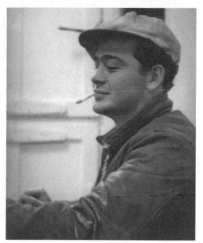

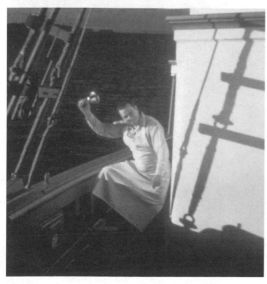

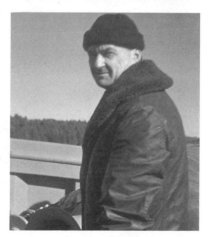

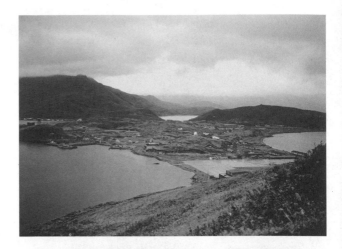

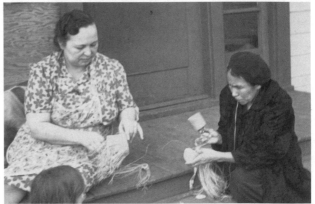

Top: Dutch Harbor.
Middle: Mrs. Hope and
Anfesia weaving Attu
baskets.
Bottom: Father
Theodosia, Russian
Orthodox Church,
Unalaska.

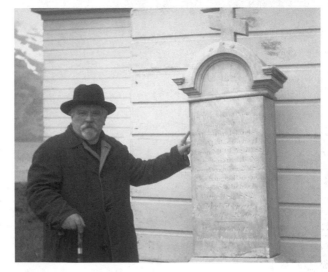

Unimak Pass had a reputation for violent currents, tide rips, and rough water. When we drew near, those affected by seasickness scurried for their bunks. The photographers looked for vantage points for interesting pictures. I made for the bridge, as I had established my interest and ability to help in the pilot house with Captain Kippola from the start of the trip.

The pass was slightly rough, but did not in any way live up to its reputation. Some of us were disappointed not to see the wild waters we had heard about, but not the captain. "We hit that just right, slack tide and good weather," he said.

Dutch Harbor
Tuesday, June 17, to Friday, June 20

Dutch Harbor had been both an Army and Navy base during World War II. Heavy, clearly visible fortifications lined the channel into the harbor. The Army and Navy were pulling out because there was no adequate airstrip. The Army was about through with its decommissioning process, and the Navy planned to leave by September.

Dr. Schwinge had spent some time in Dutch Harbor during the winter of 1946 helping the Aleuts during a diphtheria epidemic. Now she had many friends there as well as across the bay in the Native village of Unalaska. When we landed, Dr. Schwinge went up to the administration building and found an old friend, Dr. Marr.

Dr. Marr took over our "supervision." He said, "You are here just in time. We have a warehouse of medical supplies and equipment that are going to be loaded on a barge and dumped at sea. Tomorrow I will take you to the warehouse, and you can have anything you want. We hate to do this, but it costs less than moving it."

The rapidly expanding Territorial Department of Health needed just about everything that was to be dumped, but they had no money to pay for transporting the supplies. If only a way could be found to move them to Sitka, where the needs were so great! When we returned in the fall with our supplies depleted, it would be too late. They would be gone.

We had stuffed every nook and cranny on the *Hygiene*, so we could only rescue small items. Dr. Schwinge, Kitty, and I tried to choose the most needed, most expensive, and most stowable supplies and equipment from that huge warehouse. I had to pass up a beautiful microscope similar to the one I had purchased in Seattle. It broke my heart to think of it rusting on the bottom of the ocean. I did find shelves of expensive biological stains in small bottles. Some of these had been unavailable to civilian hospitals during the war, or cost so much they were used only when most urgently needed. There was no room in the clinic, but I slipped them into the bottom of my closet. Kitty and Dr. Schwinge found adhesive tape, splints, ointments, and medicines.

When we returned to the *Hygiene*, Captain Kippola informed Dr. Schwinge that Sig and Red Harris had left without a word to anyone. They had boldly lowered the launch and talked a deckhand into taking them and their gear to Unalaska. That left the *Hygiene* without a secretary, and what was worse, without an assistant engineer. We could not proceed without another engineer, and Dutch Harbor was not a place to conveniently find help of that kind.

That evening we went to Unalaska to visit Dr. Marr and his family. Dr. Schwinge explained the loss of our assistant engineer and our predicament. Dr. Marr then took us to the Bachelor Officers Quarters in Dutch Harbor, where he asked for help in finding a replacement engineer.

Through his efforts, Wendell Moore, a pleasant, middle-aged, balding man, came on board the next afternoon. Dr. Schwinge recognized him from her previous trip to Unalaska. Wendell said, "I'd like to join you but I don't want a black mark on my civil service record. I'll come if they will release me from this job." This reply left us in suspense for another day.

While we waited, I joined Dr. Schwinge when she visited Anfesia Shapsnikoff to thank her for a rare and beautiful Attu basket Anfesia had given her the day before. Dr. Schwinge asked Anfesia about her life.

Anfesia related, "I was born at Atka. My father was a Russian sailor who came on a trading boat and met my mother at Attu. They settled there, and my father lived until he was 82. My mother died of the flu in 1919." She continued, "I had three brothers and sisters, but they all died, and so have all my own children." By a process of adopting and caring for other people's children, however, she still had a large family.

A very short woman, Anfesia was scarcely four feet high because of severe kyphosis (hunched back). She and Mrs. Hope were the only two in the village who still knew how to weave the famous Attu and Atka baskets. None of the young people wished to take it up, and consequently examples of the work were very scarce. Dr. Schwinge's basket was a museum piece. Attu weaving, twisted more tightly than Atka weaving, would hold water. Dr. Schwinge persuaded Anfesia and her friend Mrs. Hope to sit on the stairs in the sunlight and demonstrate basket-making techniques while she took pictures of them.

Anfesia said she was still using grass picked on Attu before the Japanese attacked the island and captured its people on June 8, 1942. All 47 Aleuts living there were taken to Japan on the *Yaksha*. Mike Kodiakoff, the chief, died in Japan with 27 others. Fifteen were returned to Atka, not Attu. Five babies were born in Japan. One had returned, and four others were in hospitals stateside. When we left, Anfesia assured Dr. Schwinge that she and Mrs. Hope would organize the village to be ready for their X-ray survey when we returned.

While we were at the dock, the captain was having problems with the radio equipment. A Navy officer kindly offered the services of a young sailor who quickly fixed the radio, but soon all the other equipment began to blow fuses. The captain and Gus could not find the cause. Dr. Schwinge made another trip to the Bachelor Officers Quarters for help. An army electrician arrived first thing in the morning and had everything ship-shape in a couple of hours.

A short time later Wendell Moore came in and accepted the job as assistant engineer, after finally obtaining a release from his Civil Service job. It was beginning to look as though we might continue our journey as early as the next day.

That afternoon Father Theodosius, the visiting priest from the Pribilofs, invited Jessie, Kitty, Dr. Schwinge, and me to visit the church, which had a friendly and active congregation. He encouraged us to explore and take pictures. The priest had been born in Russia, in the Ukraine. He had come to the U.S. in 1910 and worked in the States, then in Alaska. In the States he had lived among Slavic people and never learned English until he was established in Unalaska during the war. As a consequence his accent was very thick, and it was hard to understand him.

The night before we left, the Coast Guard cutter *Wachussetts* pulled in. She was carrying the court party consisting of Judge Dimond and several lawyers. They would settle all the legal matters of Unalaska during their short visit.

Dr. Schwinge and I paid our last respects to Dr. Marr while the crew filled the ship's tanks with fuel and water the next morning. A nurse came running down the dock with three pile-lined Army surplus parkas. She said, "They aren't beautiful but I'll guarantee you will need them!" We thanked her for the gifts, but wondered how we would be able to use them in the middle of summer. Finally we left, lacking only a secretary, bulging with supplies, and with hearty bon voyages ringing in our ears.

Bering Sea
Friday, June 20, to Monday, June 23

In Dutch Harbor, the Aleutian Islands lived up to their reputation for cold, fog, and generally miserable weather, but while we sailed north across the Bering

Sea, we reveled in sunshine and calm seas. Saturday, June 21, was the longest day of the year. At one point Nunivak Island appeared on the distant horizon. Kidding and joking about the horrors of the Bering Sea, we spread out over the deck to soak up the sun.

So far, we were happy shipmates. Captain Kippola and Dr. Schwinge were getting along in a most amiable manner. He was a high-strung, nervous man, but very competent. Dr. Schwinge had a wonderful sense of humor and was so considerate it would have been hard to pick a fight with her. Kitty and I looked forward to the next month's work.

Captain Kippola made radio contact with Nome, and the operator promised to send messages explaining the purpose of our visits and the approximate dates of arrival to Golovnin, White Mountain, Elim, Koyuk, and to the ANS nurse at Unalakleet.

After a night of daylight, we awoke to an ocean still calm. In all directions we could see nothing but miles and miles of tranquil seas. Puffy clouds drifted across the horizon, and at one point near the Yukon Delta, shower clouds hung over the river. Early Monday morning Golovnin appeared under clear and sunny skies.

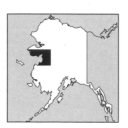

Norton Sound

Golovnin (Golovin) and White Mountain
Monday, June 23, to Monday, June 30

About 25 unpainted houses stretched in a row on a long flat sandspit. The ocean, marsh, and grass surrounding the village emphasized the vast and lonely space. Man and his works seemed very small.

A large freighter, the *Reef Knot,* lay in the outer bay unloading as we came in. Each town lightered their year's supplies to shore on barges pulled by shallow-draft tugs. The Bering Sea could be compared to a flat saucer. The beaches sloped out gradually, making it necessary for some of the larger ships to anchor so far from shore they could not see the villages they were servicing.

Rows of breakers along the shoreline in front of Golovnin looked too difficult for our motor launch to breach, so Gus rowed Kitty and Dr. Schwinge ashore to meet the schoolteachers, Mr. and Mrs. Daugherty. Victor Hill, the teacher from neighboring White Mountain, was also there. His students were helping transfer supplies from the freighter.

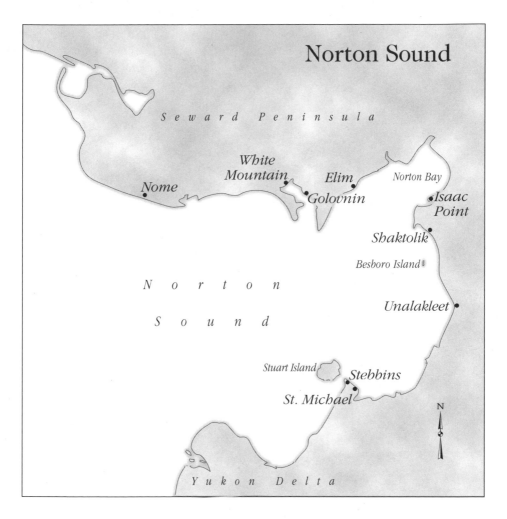

Norton Sound was our first contact with the Eskimo culture. Kayaks, dog sleds and dogs were a way of life. Night as we knew it did not exist, nor did regular hours. We were welcomed enthusiastically by the villagers, most of whom spoke some English.

A familiar problem again surfaced. We were not expected; the teachers had received no message from Nome. We had hoped that in these isolated areas, radio communication might be more dependable. Quickly the teachers adapted to the situation and made plans to transport the White Mountain villagers and vocational students down the river by barge to Golovnin on Wednesday and Thursday. We would examine the population of Golovnin immediately.

Mr. and Mrs. Daugherty were Seventh Day Adventist missionaries as well as teachers. They were fine, intelligent people who offered the schoolhouse and whatever help was needed. Dr. Schwinge decided to work ashore that day and give the crew their Sunday on Monday.

Assisted by Mrs. Daugherty, she swung into our routine in this village of 125. That evening Mr. Daugherty showed two reels of the ship's health movies with his projector. Skillfully he applied the contents of the film to the villagers' particular problems. During the film on alcoholism, he reminded the audience of a villager who drank himself to death, and of the little children who ran to the schoolhouse for protection while their parents were drinking.

In the discussion after the movie on drinking water, he commented on the "dirty well" where people had spit and thrown dirty dishes, and asked who had drunk water from it? He also asked who had drunk water from the spring, only to discover that five human bodies had escaped from their coffins and were floating on the surface.

After the movies Mr. Daugherty stood up in front of the audience and said in a Barnum and Bailey voice, "Right this way, folks, come and get your typhoid shot." The response was phenomenal. Then the enthusiastic group wanted to see the movies all over again. After that, Dr. Schwinge and Kitty made an effort to show the films before the clinics to which they applied, rather than afterward. Mr. Daugherty was pleased to learn that he could get more films from the health educator at Juneau.

In the clinic the next morning, we admired the summer parkas in which the women carried their babies. A shawl that passed under the child's bottom and across the mother's shoulder kept the infant safe and warm. The parkas were roomy, gay, and excellent windbreakers. Bright-patterned cotton material on the outside covered furry skins on the inside. Footwear was divided between shoepaks (boots with leather tops and rubber feet) and mukluks.

Many of the men at that time were lightering freight, but the two villages responded enthusiastically to our program, undoubtedly partly a reflection of the teachers' leadership. We felt good about working with the friendly Eskimos. They obviously needed our services.

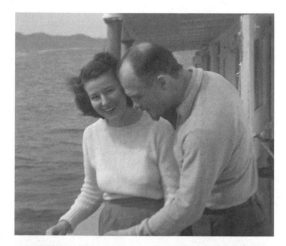

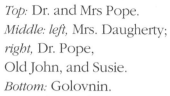

Top: Dr. and Mrs Pope.
Middle: left, Mrs. Daugherty;
right, Dr. Pope,
Old John, and Susie.
Bottom: Golovnin.

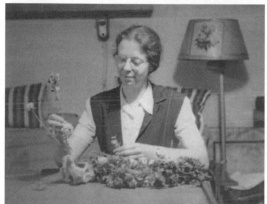

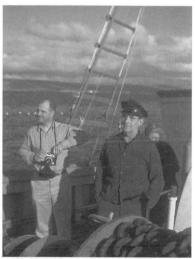

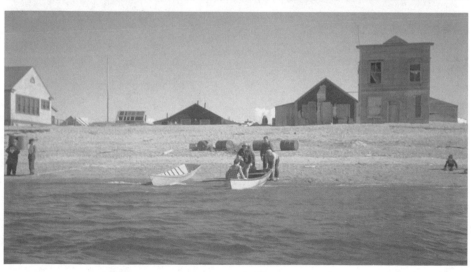

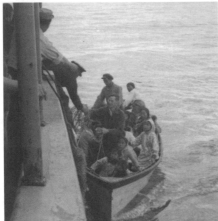

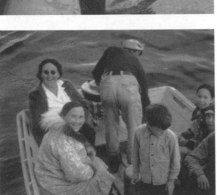

Top and middle left: Patients arriving.
Right: Golovnin beach.
Below: cleaning fish, Golovnin.

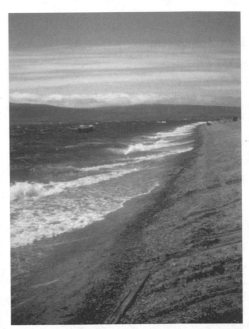

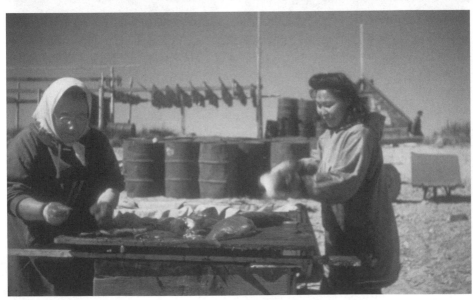

At 11 p.m. on our second day, Gus was waiting at the beach to take Dr. Schwinge, Kitty, and me back to the *Hygiene*. After a long, hard day we climbed wearily into the leaky old rowboat, ankle deep in water. Gus transported us through the surf in the little boat, poling it out 20 or 30 feet to the motor launch. Once we had clambered aboard the launch from the tipsy rowboat, we selected seats and bundled our surplus GI parkas over our heads in a futile effort to stay dry. (Now we knew why we needed them.) The launch, a fine boat on calm seas, proved a poor contrast to the local dories, which were long, narrow, and deep. They sliced through the waves and the outboard motors made it possible to run them up on the beach.

Gus started the engine in no time, and we raced for the warmth and shelter of the *Hygiene*. The four of us huddled down for the three-quarter mile ride through the waves. Halfway out, the motor stopped. Gus discovered that it was out of gas, and he had not brought an extra tank. There we sat, tired, wet, and a bit disgusted. Dr. Schwinge made a new rule that the launch should never leave the ship without an extra tank of gas and life jackets.

I helped Gus drag out the oars and we started rowing toward the village. The current was taking us away from the *Hygiene* and past the village faster than we could row. After about 15 minutes, we heard the welcome sound of an outboard motor.

A young Eskimo couple asked, "Are you taking pictures of the sunset?" Dr. Schwinge said, "I've taken pictures, but we sure do need a tow." The couple took our line and proceeded to the *Hygiene*. Tired, cold, and soggy, we finally made it to bed by midnight.

After Dr. Schwinge worked with Mrs. Daugherty for a few days, she persuaded her that she would be extremely valuable to us if she could stay until we had a new secretary. The doctor said, "You are not only a good typist and a well-organized person, but you are of even greater value because you know the people and they trust you." Mrs. Daugherty talked it over with her husband and son, who agreed that she could help out for one month.

Apparently Dr. Schwinge's wire to the Juneau office explaining Sig's and Red's departure had been ignored. She fumed, "At least they could acknowledge that they know our predicament. I hope they can get someone here in a month."

The White Mountain establishment was a vocational boarding school for Eskimo children in all grades through high school. Mr. Victor Hill, an obliging man, brought three-quarters of the villagers down the 26 miles of river to Golovnin on his boat the *San-Pan*. He made two long trips on two consecutive days, with only a few hours of sleep between them.

Arriving about 5 p.m., men, women, and children jammed the *Hygiene*. We completed the X-rays, bloods, and immunizations at 11 p.m. In the Bering Sea area, no such thing as night or regular mealtimes existed for either the Eskimos or for us. Routine hours were a luxury of the past. We felt the impact of 60 patients per day.

After five 12-hour days, during which we discovered a high incidence of TB, we were pretty well exhausted. Dr. Schwinge worked right along with Kitty and me. She was well aware of how tired we were after the long hours and did not suggest more work unless it was necessary. We each worked as hard as we could, and the cooperative atmosphere enabled us to accomplish far more than we believed possible.

Dr. Schwinge held her TB conferences. This was the time when the doctor explained the disease to each patient and answered questions they might have. Afterwards she talked with a kindly middle-aged Eskimo woman who was concerned about her eight-year-old daughter Virginia. Dr. Schwinge thought Virginia's chest looked like a reinfection type of TB, probably caused by close contact with an active case. Later Dr. Schwinge heard that Virginia's mother was treating her by putting goose-grease packs on the child's chest and other local remedies, because someone else's girl had improved with such home treatment.

The doctor was also concerned about Jennie and her family, especially her three-year-old girl. Jennie always went around with a worried expression. She was having trouble keeping up with her 17 children—the last two were twins. Her oldest daughter had been treated for gonorrhea, and Jennie wanted the three-year-old to have the treatment because she was sleeping in the same bed with her infected sister.

One of the X-ray reports was a cause for celebration. It was on a one-year-old boy whose parents had both died of TB. His foster parents, a young couple expecting their first child, had planned to give him up after their own baby was born, fearing theirs would be infected. The orphan's negative X-ray report assured him of a happy home.

By late Friday afternoon the work began to ease. Dr. Schwinge took some time off to develop the pictures she had taken. Kitty was trying to establish a series of Kodachrome slides showing prenatal and infant care similar to "It Can Be Done," the series of slides we had used in Southeast Alaska. One family in Golovnin kindly posed for her, and she was anxiously awaiting the development of the pictures.

Ashore we met a new life style. This was the country of sled dogs and sleds, some of which were meticulously crafted. The dogs were beautiful in a hungry-looking way. Each one was tied to a post about six inches in diameter and three feet high. The posts were set in clusters. I started over to pat one of the animals.

Mr. Daugherty shouted, "Susie, stop! Don't go close or put your hand out." I said, "They look pretty friendly."

He explained, "It's summertime and the dogs aren't working, so they are fed just enough to keep them alive. They aren't vicious, just starving, and they will bite."

It was kayak country also. Canvas covered some of the sleek little craft, but the most beautiful were covered with oogoruk skin (oogoruk is the Eskimo name for bearded seal) and were snowy white. A young man explained that they used the white ones for hunting on the ice.

In the summer the people lived on the sandy beach and the tundra just above it. Fishing went on constantly. The young children pulled nets attached to the shore in and out with rowboats. Women split the fish open and put them on racks to dry at the tundra's edge. These fish were to feed the dogs during the winter. The women sat on the ground near the drying racks, chatting and laughing as they worked. Children were everywhere, playing games, fishing, and having a good time in the boats and on the beach.

This happy community life was vastly different from the way people walled themselves off from one another in the cities. I mused it would be hard to be lonesome in an Eskimo village, especially in the summer. The people did not keep any sort of formal hours. Children laughed and shouted as they played throughout the night. During the day they often curled up and slept beside a boat or an oil drum until they awakened naturally. Meals seemed to be equally impromptu—people ate whenever they were hungry; their diet was mainly fish soups, wild greens, and berries.

Dr. and Mrs. Pope, the newly married dentist and his wife, a dental technician, arrived by plane late Friday afternoon. They were upset, as they had expected the Hygiene to pick them up in Nome on Sunday. When Dr. Schwinge had found they could fly to Golovnin, she asked them to do that to save the ship two days of traveling. Dr. Pope also was concerned, with reason, because none of his dental instruments or dental X-ray film had come to Nome or Golovnin. Nor did he like the arrangement of the dental clinic and immediately put Gus to work remodeling it.

We greeted the Popes cordially, but they took second place to our first mail in three weeks. Dr. Schwinge hoped that the numerous telegrams Dr. Pope had sent to Juneau about his dental instruments would remind Darrell that he had to find a secretary by the time Mrs. Daugherty's month was up. We had been devastated when Sig left, but what, at that time, had seemed a misfortune turned into something more beneficial than anyone could have anticipated. We had no idea how helpful it was to have a person on board who knew the people and their customs. Equally important a person the villagers trusted. We could not expect this to happen again.

The Popes seemed an interesting couple. He was an ex-Navy man and knew the sea. He also piloted his own plane when he was home. His wife had worked with the Red Cross in the South Pacific all through the war.

Ted Comarra, the airplane pilot who brought the Popes to Golovnin, took our messages to the Elim and Koyuk people. He suggested we should meet them at Isaac Point instead of Elim.

When Dr. Schwinge went ashore for the last picture-showing and said her thank-yous and good-byes, she heard one Eskimo woman say to another, "I'm soooo tired." She added, "They aren't the only ones— we have certainly crowded a great deal of health care and education into a very few days."

Just as we finished up the last odds and ends and secured the clinic for travel, five men who had been lightering freight up the river came in and asked for X-rays. When Dr. Schwinge heard them coughing she said, "We'd better check them." The men waited for the results—little heaps of coughing humanity collapsed on the deck. While I developed the films, Kitty gave the group sputum bottles just in case the X-rays were positive. They were, and showed a great deal of involvement. The men should have been flat on their backs in bed, but they had been doing the hardest kind of labor, packing heavy freight ashore. Dr. Schwinge said she learned an important lesson—"Never skip over someone who was working hard on the theory they wouldn't be if they were sick."

This explained the source of Virginia's TB. Her father was one of these men. Dr. Schwinge suggested that he live by himself in a small cabin away from his family, and that he take precautions when he was around them. We felt so sorry for him because he nearly cried when the doctor told him he had TB. Mrs. Daugherty knew why. She told us, "Cemetery Hill is full of his relatives!" We all hoped something could be done for him.

Paul, a full-blooded Eskimo from White Mountain, also found out that he had TB. He was greatly concerned and wanted to go to the hospital immediately. He had heard of the lack of funds in the ANS and thought if he continued longshoring, he could save enough money to get to Juneau and present himself for treatment. Dr. Schwinge thought it might be a good idea and hoped Dr. Gehrig could do something for him.

Dr. Schwinge wrote in her diary that night, "Today marks my anniversary—one year in Alaska. Right at the moment I'm so damn tired I wish I had stayed in Wisconsin. Of course, tomorrow things will be different."

We learned that the Eskimos were worried about Mrs. Daugherty and warned her about going out in *that boat*. The launch was a menace, Water could not be drained out of it, but had to be pumped out of each partition. Every wave that came over the bow drenched the occupants.

On our last trip out from Golovnin the men had safely poled the little rowboat to the launch, which we boarded. After it ran about 20 yards toward the *Hygiene*, the motor stopped. None of John's efforts brought forth any signs of life. It was dead!

John sighed, "It needs to be overhauled. Gus hasn't had time to spend on it because Dr. Pope has kept him so busy remodeling his office." There we sat. Earlier we had tried rowing but the oars were too small to be effective in the launch. We drifted helplessly through all of the Natives' fish nets. Fortunately the propeller did not become entangled.

After trying repeatedly to land, we managed to get ashore and find someone to tow us back to the *Hygiene*. Cold, wet, and disgusted, with three hours wasted on the launch, we dreaded the thought of having to travel 17 miles from the *Hygiene* to some of the Yukon delta towns. Dr. Schwinge said, "I'm glad I'll be off the boat then. I like to live—I'm too happy to die so young."

Elim to Isaac Point
Monday, June 30, to Friday, July 4

We traveled four hours to Elim, where David Saccahus, the Eskimo storekeeper, came alongside in his dory before our crew could launch the shoreboat. This smiling round-faced Native won our gratitude when he offered to ferry us back and forth between the ship and the village. We wondered if stories of our unreliable launch had been radioed ahead.

The community had a poor harbor and a desolate air. Amazingly, trees were growing along the coast, the first we had seen on this trip since we left Juneau. Fish and dogs were everywhere. A few scattered buildings, some of them with sod roofs, nestled into the landscape. The schoolhouse was in fairly good condition but was filled with broken-down furniture. David Saccahus complained that the teachers were constantly changing. They would come for a year and then leave.

Dr. Schwinge, Kitty, and I went ashore immediately to start the exam routine. Mrs. Pope came later to help Dr. Schwinge with the record-keeping. When we returned to the ship, we found Dr. Pope was taking care of the many dental emergencies by pulling teeth. He explained that it was all he could do until his instruments came. Kitty had noticed that many of the children were hanging over the ship's rail. She looked over to see what they were watching and discovered they had just left the dentist's office and were spitting blood overboard.

After supper we started to work again. In the midst of the session Kitty's normally rosy cheeks turned deathly pale and she began to shake. Dr. Schwinge checked her, discovered she had a fever and all the symptoms of flu, and sent her to bed immediately. Mrs. Daugherty filled in and did a good job taking case histories. How lucky we were to have her on board! Kitty's fever persisted, but in spite of feeling tired and achy she tried to work, until Dr. Schwinge told her to go to bed and lie down before she fell down.

Some older arthritic adults had walked nine miles to bring a group of children for their shots. All had been severely bitten by mosquitoes and hoped for relief from their aches and pains. They were disappointed when Dr. Schwinge could give them no immediate relief. Her diary entry for that day read: "Damn it, I hate to be rushed in my work. To think that the *Hygiene* spends months in Southeast villages, and these poor Eskimos get hours. According to these people, it would be safe for the *Hygiene* to travel here in June. We are a month late again."

After that entry, the weary doctor was ready for sleep. Just as she was about to crawl into her bunk, she noticed something dripping from the ceiling onto her pillow; it was coming from the batteries, and it did not smell like water. She called Dell, who was on night watch. He came down and helped her hang up a bucket. There she was, 15 minutes later, listening to the steady drip, drip, drip of battery acid over her head. She did not have to listen long, for about 12:30 a.m. the wind started to blow hard. Dr. Schwinge got up to see if everything was secure in her office, imagining view boxes bouncing around on the floor, along with my microscope.

The skipper had anchored as close to shore as possible. Our stern was in about four feet of water, a safe depth when it was calm. The wind had come up suddenly, and in a few minutes the swells were almost large enough to bounce the boat on the bottom. By 12:45 a.m. we were all up, as Captain Kippola moved to deeper water.

The motor launch was the main casualty. Early in the trip the captain had delegated the responsibility for the launch to Gus. He would be responsible for its maintenance and use. Earlier that night the deckhands had wanted to go ashore. So Gus, Mr. Moore, and Wayne lowered the boat. However, the fellows found when they were still 50 yards from the beach that the water was too shallow to continue. Therefore they came back. When the skipper suggested that they return the launch to the top deck, Gus said, "We'll need it in the morning. Might as well leave it in the water." So they left the boat out.

Then the wind came up and the *Hygiene* had to move within 10 minutes to safer waters. The captain tried to recover the launch, but the waves smashed it against the *Hygiene* and stove in one side. Gus claimed the skipper should not have tried to get it aboard then. Perhaps that was true, but the skipper countered that it never should have left the deck, and that also was true—bad judgment all the way around. None of the shore-boat decisions had been wise, including its original purchase.

The following morning Dr. Schwinge decided a dory was necessary to continue the program. She said, "I can come up with only one solution. I think that I will buy a boat and turn it over to the skipper for the rest of the voyage. Later I'll ask the Department of Health to pay me for it or maybe I'll even give it to them. I can't requisition it now, what with all the rules and regulations. This way I can get a seaworthy dory of the type we need from one of the villagers." We applauded her proposal.

We next moved to Isaac Point, a lonely hill jutting out in the water, to meet the Koyuk people. We anchored there for two and a half days waiting for them. During this time I came down with the flu.

There were few signs of life on the beach, and the sea was too rough for the people to travel. Later Dr. Schwinge learned that about 20 people had come down the river the day after we left. Most of the villagers of Koyuk could not come because the men were not at home to bring them in their boats.

Kitty and I felt our guardian angels were looking out for us, as we were too sick to work. We were grateful we could lie in bed even though it did roll.

Isaac Point to Shaktolik
Friday, July 4, to Sunday, July 6

The captain and doctor decided that unless sea conditions improved the next day, we should either move on to Shaktolik, or make use of the bad weather by returning to Golovnin to take on fuel and water from the *Square Knot*, an Alaskan steamship freighter.

The next morning the seas were still rolling, and a glance at the waves pounding the beach made it obvious that anyone on shore would find it impossible to beat through the surf and rollers out to the ship. We waited until noon, however, hoping that the waves would subside.

The exhausted Dr. Schwinge went back to bed and slept all morning, deciding that rest was more important than paperwork. Kitty and I worried about her because she had been working without a break, making major decisions, and getting very little rest. We hoped she was not coming down with the flu. Steadfastly Mrs. Daugherty plugged away at the typewriter.

That afternoon the waves continued to crash on the beach, and we moved to Shaktolik, where conditions were no better. We anchored less than a mile from the shore, and the captain and doctor were able to make radio contact with Mr. Simon Newcomb, the schoolteacher. He suggested that the heavy surf on the unprotected shore might be too rough for our small boat to attempt a landing; he and the mayor of the village would come out with the census as soon as conditions allowed. Again we wondered if the "Tundra Telegraph" had spread word of the misadventures of our launch.

Just after supper, we saw a dory with four men plunging through the surf. We welcomed them aboard and enjoyed meeting Mr. Newcomb, a well-educated man with an old-world courtesy. He and his wife had been ANS teachers in the Bering Sea area since 1939. An anthropologist, he was collecting Eskimo stories, but commented that he had been so busy teaching he hadn't had much time for his collection.

Optimistically, they planned to bring the people out the next day for their X-rays. Dr. Schwinge hoped we could finish our routine in the next two or three days. Then the *Hygiene* could meet the *Square Knot* at Golovnin before proceeding to Unalakleet.

It was the Fourth of July. To celebrate, Mrs. Daugherty showed us her slides of the people of Gambell on St. Lawrence Island celebrating their Fourth of July with jumping games, tug of war, blanket tossing, and seal races. Some of us had a few nostalgic moments when we thought of our Fourth of July celebrations at home.

She went on to tell us about the Russian prisoner who escaped from Siberia with his six-year-old son. This case was once considered at the highest level by the intelligence agencies of several nations. Minikov, the Russian escapee, had been educated at the University of Moscow and was a brilliant engineer. He had traveled with the Soviet Navy and knew the Russian military installations in Siberia, as well as secret police operations.

Unfortunately, the wrong person heard him suggest that the Russians did not have much freedom in their country, so he was sent to Siberia to install fortifications, after which he was slated for the hangman's noose. While in Siberia he built his own little boat, took his son, and fled to St. Lawrence Island, where he arrived in very poor condition. The Daughertys nursed him back to health, but were unable to understand him until an interpreter Mr. Daugherty had requested was flown in by the FBI.

Minikov cooperated with the FBI and Army Intelligence and gave such accurate information about Russia that it was said he saved several thousand American lives. The U.S. government gave him naturalization papers and moved him to the States. Mr. Daugherty's sister was caring for his son. Just a few weeks after he and his son were removed, some Russians came snooping for information. Mr. Daugherty got the villagers together, and the group decided to treat the Russians courteously, but give them no information about anything. It was a ticklish diplomatic matter for the U.S. government, since we were still uneasy allies with the Soviets. This was as close as any of us had been to diplomatic intrigue.

Mrs. Daugherty explained that she and her husband Frank knew that teaching the Eskimos was a worthwhile accomplishment because both children and adults were so eager to learn. The village of Gambell on St. Lawrence Island was an example. Before the Daughertys arrived, most of the children had not been to school. Now, except for the very old, every person could read and write.

Mr. Daugherty, whose skills included wiring and plumbing, thought that the people should have electric lights. Most white people tried to discourage him: "It can't be done. The Natives can't handle machinery—the diesels will be of no value—broken down all of the time. Besides, the expenses will break the village for years to come."

But Mr. Daugherty claimed that anyone could be trained to run a diesel. He called the village council together. They decided to install a diesel engine for an electric plant to light the village. The project was completely paid for in three years, and the Eskimos maintained it themselves.

Then the Daughertys said to themselves, "How can we expect these people to keep clean when they have to walk all the way to the river and back for water?"

They dug a well and fortunately found water under the site of the future school. A heating system, community shower, laundry, and, believe it or not, flush toilets were installed. It showed what ingenuity and faith could do.

On July 5, we were rested and ready for a good day's work, but the surf was still so high that the people could not get off the beach in their dories. There we sat and rolled, with everyone growing more impatient by the hour.

Finally the skipper and the doctor decided that Shaktolik would have to wait while we went to Golovnin to meet the *Square Knot*. Water had become the most precious commodity on shipboard. Captain Kippola asked each of us to use no more than one small washbasin per day. The new water tanks installed in Juneau just before we went north were a big mistake. They were built with the wrong kind of metal, and the water in them was so rusty it was almost unusable. I wrote to my mother, "I'm dirty, my hair is dirty and so are most of my clothes and the ship's linens. There isn't a thing I can do about it until we get more water. At least we are all in the same boat, except for Mrs. Pope, who takes showers and washes her hair. She looks clean and smells good, but everyone avoids her and she can't understand why."

We arrived at Golovnin about 5 p.m. and took on fuel but were extremely disappointed to find we could not get water. The *Square Knot* still had a long voyage ahead and had to conserve its own water. The captain took us on a tour of his ship and offered us each a drink of water, not exactly what we had been anticipating. He suggested to Captain Kippola that he go across to the stream at Golovnin. It was the one place in Norton Sound where we could get within two-tenths of a mile of fresh water. Captain Kippola could then have the crew scrub out the life boat, fill it with water by buckets, tow it to the *Hygiene* and pump the water into our tanks.

After filling the fuel tanks, Captain Kippola rushed over to the stream. By then it was 1 a.m. and nearly dark, so he decided to sleep before rewatering. That was a mistake. In the morning the sea was so rough that the waves would have washed salt water into the fresh water being towed in the life boat.

Dr. Schwinge and the captain decided to return to Shaktolik rather than wait for the wind to die down. They radioed the Newcombs to have their people ready to board for X-rays at 3 p.m., or any time thereafter that sea conditions would permit.

Shaktolik
Sunday, July 6, to Wednesday, July 9

Although we were still unwashed and disappointed, a brief break in the weather enabled us to X-ray most of the population with the help of Mr. and Mrs. Newcomb. As usual, the program moved more smoothly when those who knew the village people were present. We continued with the clinic procedures despite growing seas. The place smelled like wet reindeer, and all the children were crying. It was the noisiest bunch that had yet come aboard, and we soon found out why. The poor tots were seasick. The boat kept rocking, and they would howl, and all of a sudden they would vomit. The deckhands mopped busily and hoped this would not become normal procedure in the Bering Sea.

By 11 p.m. the water became so rough that it was too dangerous for the small boats to go back and forth. We had X-rayed most the village and could finish most of the remaining work on shore if necessary. During the night we rolled so violently that it was impossible to sleep or read; we fought just to stay in our bunks. As the wind showed no sign of abating in the morning, Captain Kippola ran to hide in the lee of Besboro Island, 10 miles away. At least we could spend the day catching up on the record work after the battering we had taken during the night. It was heavenly to be in the lee after the violent rolling we had just experienced.

After supper Dr. Pope, Del, Wayne, and I rowed the skiff to a sandspit about a mile away. As we approached we could see movement on the end of the spit. It became apparent that a huge herd of seals was living there. When we came close, the guards lifted their heads and watched nervously. Some of the more wary creatures waddled awkwardly closer to the water. We rowed to the main island, hoping to sneak up on them by land. I decided against walking out the spit, since it was only six feet wide in many places and the tide was coming in. I did not want to be marooned out there. The others approached cautiously, but soon the large herd slid into the sea like a splashing wave.

The island was a giant bouquet; flowers covered the ground like a carpet. While I waited for the others to return from the spit, I picked bouquets for every room on the ship. Then, because the wind was still howling and it was spitting rain occasionally, I built a small fire. When Dr. Pope returned, he made it into a large one, but we had neglected to bring any food, so it did not do much except add to the atmosphere.

On our return we found that Dr. Schwinge had worried about our going so far in the small rowboat. She had hoped our huge fire was not a signal for help. Later in the evening, after spending the day working on records, Mrs. Daugherty showed more of her slides and told us more stories of her many years with the Eskimos.

She told of the woman who came to her and said that Mrs. Daugherty was named wrong—she should call herself Mrs. Dirty. Mrs. Daugherty was flabbergasted, for she spent many an hour cleaning. Patiently, she asked the woman, "Why?" The Eskimo said, "You always cleaning, and never come outdoors and see the geese flying or watch the sunsets."

She told us that on St. Lawrence Island, many of the small school children would almost faint about 11 a.m. because of insufficient breakfasts. This had inspired her to organize a group of the older girls to serve food in the school-house to all of the children.

During the night the wind died and the seas subsided. We rushed back to Shaktolik to continue our work between storms. As soon as we returned, the men took the doctor and Kitty ashore for TB conferences. The villagers swarmed around them and introduced many people who had arrived from fish camps and had not yet been X-rayed. I was kept busy on the ship. It was a beautiful day, and Dr. Schwinge had hoped that she could finish the TB conferences and go for a walk and take pictures. With the many new arrivals who needed her attention, she worked instead.

Some of the village men helped the crew get water from the river. That enabled us to continue working for a while. Lack of water had become a crisis. We began to fear that only a small portion of our program would be completed if we couldn't get water and the weather didn't improve.

One Eskimo man and his little boy flew in from Haycock. This man was very concerned about the little fellow, for he had just had a convulsion two days previously. The child's mother was a known active case of TB, and the man wanted to make sure that he and his son were not infected too. While the doctor read the X-rays the man watched the movie on syphilis. When it was over he dashed down to ask her about that, since he said that at one time he had been treated for syphilis, and now he wanted to know if he was all right.

The ANS nurse serving the area had done an excellent job of teaching home care. Kitty was impressed when she observed a 10-year-old boy with a severe case of TB following the nurse's recommendations. He had been given his own bed and a cupboard for his dishes and belongings. When he was up, he carried his "spit can" wherever he went. Equally impressive was the midwife's demonstration of her technique of delivering babies. She went through each step of a delivery using a fur parka as the mother. The arms of the parka became the mother's legs, and a pair of fur mittens represented the baby and placenta.

My sanitation report described the precautions the people of the village had taken to protect their drinking water—precautions we had not seen in other communities. Shaktolik was about 12 years old. Situated on a low, narrow spit between Norton Sound and the Shaktolik River, it consisted of 20 houses for the 100 inhabitants. The ANS teachers had advised and supervised the village builders throughout the town's construction. Lumber had been obtained from old Fort St. Michael, so the houses were larger and sturdier than those in some of the other communities. About half the dwellings had privies built to drain into Golovnin Bay. The drinking water was carried from the Shaktolik River in buckets, and town law was that refuse went into the bay and never into the

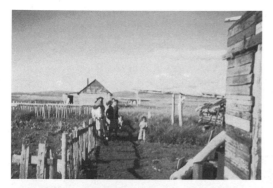

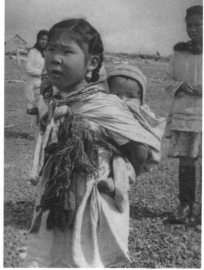

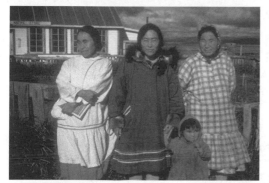

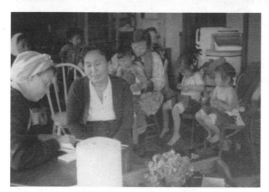

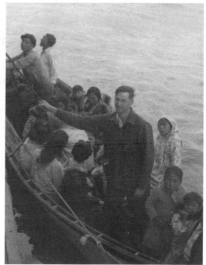

Left, top to bottom: Shaktolik garden; Shaktolik women; a full waiting room; leaving Shaktolik. *Right: above,* little girl carrying baby; *below,* Mr. Newcomb bringing patients.

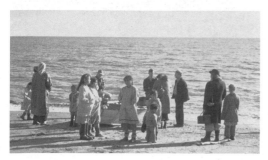

Top: left, laundry day;
right, Mr. Berry and his tomatoes.
Bottom: Unalakleet garden.

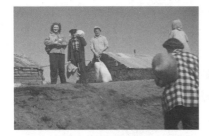

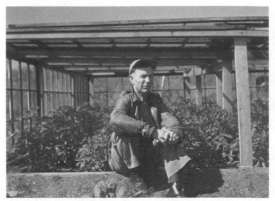

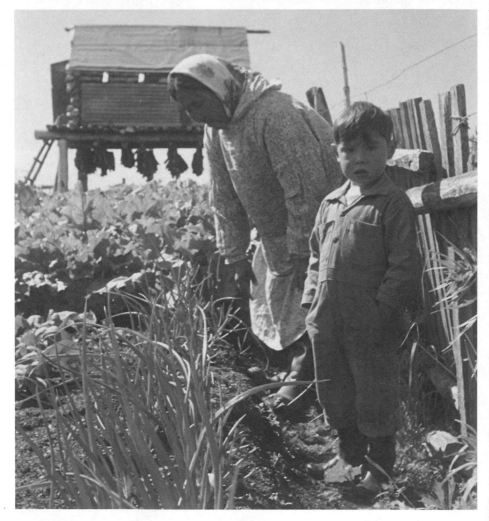

river. The dog barns were on the bay side of the town, and all dogs were chained. The dog trail went fairly close to the river, but did not enter or cross it.

In the winter, water was obtained from river ice or holes in the ice. Refuse was taken out onto the bay ice to go to sea. Mr. Newcomb had no reports of typhoid fever and only three intestinal disturbances that spring. No clam beds existed at that location, although clams were sometimes found when the wind blew the water out of the bay. This village had the best sanitation setup we had seen in the Bering Sea. Some small gardens were in evidence but Mr. Newcomb explained that the soil was too sour for them to be very successful.

The people were friendly and eager to come to the *Hygiene*. Some had traveled 20 miles to notify families at the fish camp so they could participate. Many of the older people, particularly the women, needed interpreters. It was difficult to understand them and to know if they understood what we said to them.

After finishing the X-rays, I had a chance to go ashore. The striking feature of this village was the large number of babies. Nearly every woman, from eight-year-olds up to little wizened grandmothers, had a baby on her back. Some of the babies seemed nearly as big as the person carrying them. The sunshine made it an opportune time for picture-taking. One old man with an interesting face had apparently been photographed in the past, and when I pointed to him and then my camera, he grinned broadly and snapped into a rigid pose, not even breathing. It spoiled his natural look, but he was most pleased with himself. Few of the Eskimos spoke English, so sign language was the only way to communicate.

Unalakleet
Wednesday, July 9, to Thursday, July 10

We sailed to Unalakleet in fine weather and anchored there about 10 p.m. Again the waves were larger than the skiff could handle, and with the launch smashed, we were dependent on the village people for transportation. Captain Kippola tried unsuccessfully to make radio contact. John and Gus agreed that somehow they would find a dory in town the next day.

The original reason for this stop was to pick up Miss Hankins, the ANS nurse. We were not planning to work or to get mail, although a package of dental film was waiting for Dr. Pope—but again, no dental instruments.

In the morning Mr. Berry, the schoolteacher, made several trips to take us to town. He showed us his garden and took us to the store for fresh supplies. He and his wife invited Dr. Schwinge for dinner. She reported that after some conversation to and fro about the program of the *Hygiene* and the way we worked with the Alaska Native Service, he agreed to give her a dory (he had six of them) if she would pay him for the labor which he had put into the boat. They both agreed that any problems between the departments could best be straightened out in Juneau. She paid him $40.80 for repairs he had made, and planned to turn the bill in to Dr. Albrecht. A boat was necessary to fulfill the program, and now we had a good one.

Unalakleet was an oasis of cleanliness. Six of us gathered everyone's sacks of dirty clothes and linens and took them to the town's wash-house, which also boasted showers and lots of hot water. There we did a gargantuan wash. After the long water shortage, the big tubs of soapy water released all inhibitions, and we acted like five-year-olds, decorating one another with soapsuds and having soapy water fights. The wash-house rang with laughter. It was amazing how little it took to have a good time. The sun was out and a stiff wind blowing, so the first loads were dry before the next were ready to hang out. We were all able to take showers, shampoo, wear clean clothes and make our beds with fresh linens. It was wonderful to be clean!

The Eskimos proudly showed us their beautifully kept vegetable gardens. They even had corn and tomatoes, which unfortunately were not ready to pick. The growing season started late, but once it began, the 24-hour sunlit days produced rapid growth and vegetables of great size. Only the lettuce and rhubarb were ready to harvest. Jessie bought 40 pounds of each. We could have easily eaten double that amount. The fresh food was so tasty it disappeared in a couple of days.

At last Dr. Schwinge had a chance to get out and take pictures. She captured the children in their 4-H gardens. She had always associated 4-H clubs with Wisconsin boys and girls, but now she knew of one in Unalakleet. She took photos of older Eskimo women gutting fish, making mukluks, and hoeing gardens, as well as the village with its windmills which charged battery sets for radios. These made interesting shots, as did the dogs, the fish drying, and the sod-roofed houses.

She hoped the pictures of our group from the *Hygiene* trudging ashore laden with large sacks of laundry and big boxes of soap, with all the children and dogs of the village following us, would turn out well. It was quite a sight too when she returned to the ship. Every available mast and line was covered with shirts and trousers fluttering in the breeze. The warm sunshine on the gently rolling green hills, with blue sky and white fluffy clouds overhead, gave Unalakleet a beauty similar in many respects to that of the rolling plains of the States.

Miss Hankins, the nurse who was to come with us, was a humorous, rather plump blond. She was friendly and easy to get along with, which meant a lot aboard ship. Her territory included St. Michael and Stebbins.

St. Michael and Stebbins
Friday, July 11, to Sunday, July 13

St. Michael, our next stop, exuded history. From the time of Russia's first colonization it had been an important site for access to the interior. Here priests, traders, and cargo had been transferred from oceangoing craft to shallow draft boats plying the Yukon River.

Approximately 150 Eskimos lived on the tundra above the wrecks of the famed Yukon River sternwheeled boats that still littered St. Michael's beach. Numerous barracks connected by boardwalks gave evidence of the U.S. Army's presence from the early 1900s until the 1920s. The boardwalks had been necessary to keep pedestrians from sinking up to their knees in the tundra mud. Mr. Brown, one of the residents of the town, said the Army had given permission to the ANS to use the barracks as they desired. In spite of this, the once booming center of trade proved to be somewhat of a ghost town.

While Dr. Schwinge was ashore, she took advantage of a break to visit the white trader, Herb Johnson, and his wife. She asked them about the possibility of getting water for the *Hygiene*. Again we were using the rusty, good-for-nothing water, and it was almost depleted. We were averaging just 11 gallons per person per week.

Mr. Johnson explained that their unique source of fresh water was a spring in the bottom of the ocean. At high tide, salt water covered the spring, but we could obtain the precious fresh water at low tide. He offered to bring his barge to the ship about 4 p.m. to pick up the crew and to help them fill all our barrels. Dr. Schwinge thought he was most kind—and his wife baked us delicious apple pies.

Herb's store was a jumble of Eskimo baskets and poorly carved ivory. In the back was a shortwave AC-DC battery radio (Zenith Trans-oceanic), just what Dr. Schwinge wanted. When she saw it and realized that it was $15 less than the identical model I had purchased at Kake, she bought it immediately. She was so starved for good music and up-to-date news that the price of $120 no longer mattered.

The teachers, Paul Ivanoff and his wife, were Eskimos. They graciously extended all the help they could, including the services of their teenage son

Johnny, who provided transportation. Gus made a deal with Mr. Ivanoff. He traded him our old launch engine for a new outboard motor. Now we could use the new dory. Dr. Schwinge allowed, "Gus is quite the trader. In a way, it was a blessing that the small boat was destroyed. Now we have a seaworthy boat and motor, and all for $40." I thought that Gus wasn't the only good trader—Dr. Schwinge would be hard to beat.

St. Michael was a more difficult town to work in than the preceding villages because we had to do all the work through interpreters. The blank expressions on the people's faces left us wondering if we were being understood. Kitty laughed when she told of her experience with an elderly Eskimo woman who had listened, with a totally expressionless face, to her explanation of how people with TB should sleep away from others and not kiss anyone. She asked this older lady to repeat what she had just told her. The woman just shook her head and said, "I can't." Then she grinned and said, "Good thing I got no boyfriend."

I described my problem at the X-ray machine. "I tell them to take a deep breath and hold it and nothing happens, they don't move even when the interpreter tells them. I know they are frightened by the X-ray machine, but it just is not possible to comfort each person, especially through an interpreter who is not too sure of the situation himself." It was important, where most of the people don't speak or understand English, for the teachers or village leaders to explain ahead of time to their townspeople what the *Hygiene* was doing and why.

The first water trip with Mr. Johnson brought us a mere 300 gallons, which I chlorinated. Earlier Dr. Schwinge had been truly angry when the men had put water in one of the tanks while we were ashore, then conveniently forgot to mention it. The men still believed that I was ruining good water every time I added the chlorine. Dr. Schwinge showed that she could lose her temper over that kind of monkey business. She told them she did not have time to take care of an epidemic of gastrointestinal diseases on the ship.

Mr. Johnson and the *Hygiene* crew carried on the water operation throughout our stay in St. Michael and managed to collect about 1000 gallons. I continued chlorinating the water and, for once, no one commented on it.

One afternoon a woman came running into the shore clinic. Upset and breathless she panted, "A boy is having a fit."

Mrs. Ivanoff pushed her away and said, "The boy is always having fits." Dr. Schwinge found out that the lad had been swimming in a pond with some other children, had an epileptic seizure, and went under. No one knew how long he had been under water. He was not breathing at the time they brought him in. We started artificial respiration immediately. (Artificial respiration in those days was done by straddling the patient, sitting back on your haunches and coming forward with a push on the rib cage while reciting "Out goes the bad air, in comes the good," for rhythm.)

Dr. Schwinge, Johnny Ivanoff, Kitty, and I took turns trying to resuscitate him. Several times we thought he took a breath, so we kept working on him, hoping for another. After what seemed like forever, Dr. Schwinge pronounced him dead. We returned to the ship exhausted and sad that our efforts had failed. Later we found out that he had apparently been under water for some time before his mother found him. We discussed writing to the American Red Cross to recommend that they try to establish first aid programs in the rural villages of Alaska.

On our last day, some of the people from Stebbins, a small undeveloped village, hiked the six miles to St. Michael to attend clinics. We were appalled at the number of severe cases of TB in these two communities. Dr. Schwinge and Kitty thought Miss Hankins should stay at St. Michael for follow-up work, but Miss Hankins elected to return to Unalakleet.

We left that evening loaded with Stebbins people. A large bonfire on the beach in front of their town guided us to a point where their small boats could retrieve them. Fortunately the weather was good.

At St. Michael a major crew problem developed. Wayne, one of the deckhands, was on the lazy side. He had talked back frequently to the captain, who finally ran out of patience and fired him. This was a normal procedure, except that Wayne was stranded in St. Michael.

A second problem reared its ugly head when the captain hired Johnny Ivanoff to replace Wayne. Johnny had not only been helpful ferrying people back and forth, but he had been an excellent interpreter and a willing assistant. We on the medical staff thought Johnny would be an excellent addition. The fact that the captain would leave Wayne in an isolated place like St. Michael with no way out, however, upset the crew. And they did not want to share their quarters with a "dumb, dirty Eskimo."

We couldn't believe our ears. Johnny was cleaner than any of us at that point. Kitty heatedly pointed out to Gus that Johnny not only spoke his Native language but spoke English fluently. Kitty asked, "Can you speak his language?"

Gus replied, ignoring her question "Well, the whole crew is planning to walk off in Nome."

Dr. Schwinge met with the captain and persuaded him to take Wayne as far as Nome. In the meantime, Johnny's sunny personality, humor, and above all his zeal in making our program work soon earned him the respect of the crew members.

At the same time we on the medical staff had our own problem, in the form of Dr. Pope, the dentist. He was a rather authoritarian, dogmatic man of 40 who was often hostile to our 26-year-old female physician. He played games to break up the cooperative relationship that she had with the captain. Even though we were exhausted, Dr. Pope was not able to destroy the loyalty that the captain, the crew, and her staff had for Dr. Schwinge. She provided the leadership and inspiration that enabled us to work without regard for hours or meals. The weather alone had dictated our schedules. Frequently storms calmed down by about 10 p.m. When that happened, we X-rayed either until the work was done or another storm came. The constant rolling during the storms made a good rest impossible, but I wrote to my mother, "I wouldn't miss this experience for anything."

St. Michael to Gambell
Sunday, July 13, to Wednesday, July 16

On our way to Nome, where we planned to pick up mail, dental instruments, and drop off Miss Hankins and Wayne, rough seas forced us into the protection of Golovnin Bay for the night. The storm continued through the next day, Sunday. After a brief consultation, the captain and doctor declared it a day of rest. How wonderful it felt to move and sleep without constantly bracing against the roll—to rest in peace! Mostly the wind was our enemy. This time it gave us a brief respite from work and the constant rolling.

Early Monday morning we again plowed through the rough seas towards Nome. There we joined the mail boat and a small tug hanging on their anchors in the shelter of Sledge Island, which lay a short distance off the coast. In addition, three large freighters lay chugging in the roadstead. Nome had no dock, and all freight and passengers had to be lightered to a small boat harbor built into the exposed coastline.

We waited through the day, hoping the storm would subside. About 5 p.m. it became apparent that the weather and seas were not improving, so Captain Kippola sent Miss Hankins, Wayne, and our outgoing mail over to the mail boat *Kotzebue*, to be ferried into Nome when the wind died. We started across the Bering Sea headed for Gambell, on St. Lawrence Island.

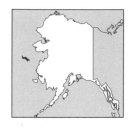

St. Lawrence Island

Gambell
Wednesday, July 16, to Monday, July 21

Again the wind howled and the waves pounded us as we crossed from Nome to St. Lawrence Island during the night, but when we pulled into the lee of the island, the seas quieted. Captain Kippola dropped the anchor a half mile from shore about 8 a.m. After he scanned the shore with binoculars, he decided that the surf breaking on the beach was too high even for the new dory. He contacted the teachers by radio and asked them to come to us if it was possible. While we waited, we went out on deck to take pictures.

This was the bleak Arctic. The town sat on a large, flat gravel point, with a high, barren bluff behind and cold gray water on three sides. The aspect, with no trees and little vegetation, was forbidding. It was *cold*—we wore mittens, hats, heavy jackets, and scarves—and this was the middle of July.

Soon a skin boat full of Eskimo traders and the schoolteacher, Mr. Reed, approached the ship. Each of the Natives had a little flour sack full of ivory, leather balls, and all kinds of knickknacks for sale. While Mr. Reed conferred with us, the men set up interesting small displays on the deck to tantalize us. Mrs. Daugherty curbed our temptation by advising us not to buy anything until we had seen what was available on shore.

Dr. Schwinge told Mr. Reed she would like to start the X-ray program that afternoon, but while they were talking, the wind picked up, and the Eskimo boatmen said it was too rough to bring the women and children to the *Hygiene*. Instead they suggested that we go ashore in their large umiak, to start our introductory work in the village. The adventure of riding in a skin boat excited me, and I confidently dropped from the ship's ladder into the fragile skin boat, tossing about on eight foot waves. I felt secure with the 12 Eskimos armed with paddles and two outboard motors.

When the umiak was fairly close to shore where the waves were beginning to break, the motor stopped. The boat swung sideways and sat on the curling crest of an eight-foot wave. The Eskimos, shouting in Yupik, grabbed their paddles, and we flew sideways toward the beach, the roar of the surf pounding our ears. My confidence in the Eskimo crew plummeted. What a time for the motor to stop! I envisioned the surf turning us over, and slamming us on the beach, and ruining my new camera. I noticed Kitty and the doctor clutched their medical bags.

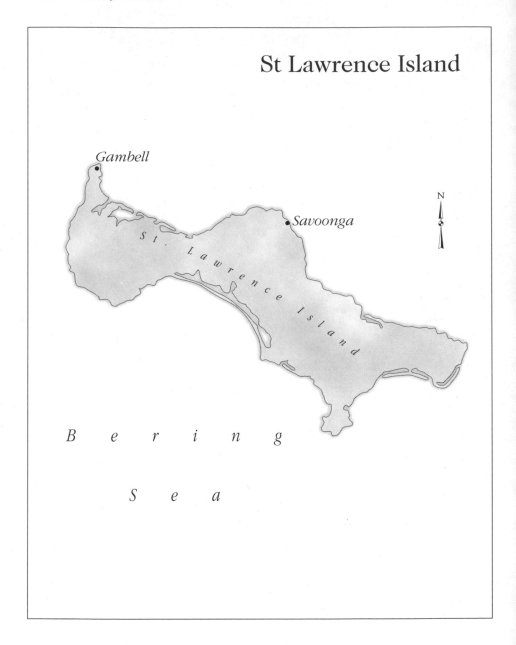

St Lawrence Island

Gambell

Savoonga

N

St. Lawrence Island

B e r i n g

S e a

Separation from the rest of Alaska and the U.S. was evident in the villages of St. Lawrence Island. Our interpreter had great difficulty with the dialect. Russia was closer than Alaska, and many of the residents had relatives in Siberia, but could no longer visit back and forth. The islanders appeared to be happy people who were genuinely concerned about their neighbors.

Suddenly the boat was high, dry, and right-side-up on the steep gravelly beach. The wave rolled back; the Eskimos, still shouting, jumped out and quickly pulled the umiak out of reach of the next wave. I started to breathe again.

After all was secure, one of the Eskimo men who spoke English told us this was standard procedure; they cut the motor intentionally and all the shouting was a normal part of deciding which wave to ride in on. If only we had understood what they were saying, we would not have been frightened. I now empathized with our scared patients who stood in front of the whirring X-ray machine, holding their breath, not knowing if they would be hurt and not understanding a word of what we said.

The umiaks were seaworthy large open boats made of a light framework of branches or animal ribs lashed with thongs and covered with walrus hide. The ropes were of walrus hide also. Many sealskin pokes lay around. The Eskimos took a complete skin, tied off all the openings and then blew it up like a balloon. They used these pokes as bumpers between two boats, as life preservers, as floats to tie onto spears in walrus hunting, and also as rollers to roll the boats up on the beach. In summer the women collected berries and stored them in the pokes, thus providing a source of vitamin C during the long winter.

People standing along the way smiled and greeted us as we walked to the town. We shook hands with everyone as we passed. The Eskimo women wore bright, printed fabric summer parkas, with the fur on the inside, and mukluks on their feet. The hoods were up against the cold, and often the women had their arms inside the body of the parka. In the winter they wore a second parka over the summer one. The winter parka was lined with fabric and had the fur on the outside. Many of the hoods were trimmed with beautiful black fur. Dr. Schwinge asked one of the girls what kind of animal the black fur came from. "It is rabbit fur dyed black, we get it from Seattle." The thicker and blacker the ruff, the more stylish it was. White cotton work gloves and a cotton drawstring bag completed the outfit. Mrs. Daugherty pointed out to us that each village had its own unique and traditional rows of rickrack trim of various colors near the hem of the parkas.

I spent the afternoon filling out the 350 X-ray cards. Kitty and Dr. Schwinge explained our various procedures to a group of high school girls who would be our interpreters. That evening as we trudged through the gravel to meet our dory on the beach, we passed many tethered hungry sled dogs. These Siberian huskies watched us with pale-blue eyes, some so pale as to look almost white. We were tired, hungry, and cold from the fierce wind that blew constantly, and we looked forward to the relative comfort of the ship and a good hot dinner, but no dory awaited us. Kitty pointed to a small boat drifting toward the Siberian coast.

"Could that be our boat?" she asked. The Eskimos on the beach talked and gestured in excitement, but we couldn't understand them. Soon Kitty's question was answered when we saw two crew members on the *Hygiene* haul up the anchor, and the ship went to rescue the dory, which had floated past the protection of the island into very rough water.

We shivered on the beach while we watched the men haul up the drifting dory, return to the shelter of the island, and re-anchor. We hoped our dory would now retrieve us, but no one came. An hour later an Eskimo who spoke English came down from the village and offered to take us back to the ship. Gratefully we accepted his offer. He warned us that the the dory should always be equipped with two working motors. When they dropped us off at the ship, the Eskimos allowed that the water was calm enough to safely bring the families out for their X-rays that evening.

Dr. Schwinge told them we would start to X-ray as soon as the boats could return. Then we heard what had happened to our dory. Inexplicably, the motor had stopped, and the wind had blown the helpless men past the shelter of the point. Captain Kippola went to rescue them, and while they were hauling up the dory, a tremendous wave rolled the *Hygiene* so far over that the galley stove blew up and so did our hot meal. The dory survived.

After peanut butter sandwiches, we started to work on the first 100 patients. Again we encountered the dismal results of ministering to seasick Eskimos. Soon all the wastebaskets were filled, and the deckhands were busy emptying them and mopping the decks, a job they did not appreciate. About midnight the wind rose again, and our crew faced the daunting task of returning the women and children to the umiaks.

The umiaks were tied to the side of the *Hygiene* where the ladder was attached. There they rose and fell on the waves, sometimes as much as six or seven feet. To get from the *Hygiene* down into an umiak required agility and speed to time the maneuver to the waves. In order to help the women and children, two of our crew members stood on a narrow ironbark rub-rail on the outside of the ship on either side of the ladder. They held a stanchion with one hand; then with the other hand, each would get a firm grip under the arm of a woman, many of whom showed the effects of their diet of blubber. Quickly the men would ease, or sometimes drop, the woman into the waiting skin boat the moment it rose on the top of a swell. They tossed the smaller children into the arms of the men below. So ended our first day in Gambell on St. Lawrence Island.

We continued our program, doing most of the work on board ship between 10 p.m. and 3 a.m., about the only time the wind took a rest. Besides seasickness, the rolling caused the women and children to lose their balance as they walked across the open space to the X-ray machine. I practically had to carry them across and back. This was quite tiring, because I had a little trouble with my own balance.

Adelinda Womkon and Della Apposingok, two bright and intelligent teenagers who spoke English well, had volunteered their services as errand runners, interpreters, or anything else they could do. Johnny Ivanoff, who had been such a good interpreter at St. Michael, could barely understand the dialect spoken on St. Lawrence Island. This was a surprise, although we had to admit Texans did not sound like New Yorkers either.

The microscope fascinated Adelinda and Della. I showed them TB germs and blood cells while I explained some of the techniques I used. We were confident that with Dr. Schwinge's and Kitty's talks and films, these alert teenagers gained a better understanding of the nature of a communicable disease like tuberculosis, and how it was spread. Eagerly they made plans for schooling to become nurses. We hoped the inspiration would last and the girls could find educational funds. The greatest obstacle would be their fathers, who did not want them to leave home.

Nurses who understood the Eskimo culture and special problems were urgently needed. For instance, canned baby food was not available, so the mother chewed the food and then gave it to the baby. She might or might not have an active case of TB to give to the baby also. Even here cleanliness was another problem not too easily understood until one saw that some villagers had to lug all their water, sometimes as far as half a mile, to their homes. This chore was not conducive to unnecessary (or even necessary) washing. Many of the people had lice in their hair, but just to delouse and wash the hair was not sufficient. The fur on the parka was also infected.

Jimmy, a town resident, demonstrated the intelligence and ability of these Natives. He had taken care of the town's dental needs to a large extent, doing excellent work in extractions, fillings, and monthly examinations on the schoolchildren. The Coast Guard dentists, who called on the town every year, had taught him basic dentistry procedures and had sent him much equipment.

Aided by his wife, Dr. Pope, who still had very few instruments, pulled teeth for two hours, his solution to dental problems. This practice left a large number of young teenagers with no front teeth and no hope of getting any. They might have been better off if the work had been left to Jimmy.

Many of Gambell's buildings were Siberian-style houses constructed with eight sides, giving them a round appearance. Sealskins were tacked to the roofs to dry. The entry was a small, raised door in the wall, about two feet above floor level, which in the winter allowed easier access and protection from blizzards and snowdrifts. The entry room, about two-thirds of the house, was similar to an enclosed back porch. Tools and outer clothes hung on the walls. Birds and fish dangled from the rafters to dry.

We entered the living quarters, a much smaller room, through another tiny raised door. A few of the houses had beds, but most of the Eskimos sat or lay on the floor. They slept on beds of furs, skins, and a few blankets. These were rolled up along one wall during the day. The residents built shelves into the walls. Electric stoves, a few washing machines, and many radios enabled the people of the village to take advantage of their power plant. We saw no electric refrigerators. Some of the houses were spotless, others not.

Mrs. Daugherty had found a lovely pair of spring dress-up mukluks for me, and I started to wear them immediately. The soles were of bearded seal, or oogoruk, and the tops of sealskin dyed red with willow bark were soft as a handkerchief. White sealskin straps tied them on my feet, and white reindeer hair decorated the tops. With the addition of a felt insole, the mukluks were warm and comfortable and weighed practically nothing, nor did they have an odor.

Kitty, too, had invested $20 in fur mukluks. Hers had reindeer uppers trimmed with beadwork around the cuff. They were a little tight but soon stretched to a comfortable fit. Once she got used to walking with no heels, she found that she had a sense of buoyancy, no doubt what God had intended. We chuckled when several Eskimo women asked if they could buy our new-found mukluks.

The discovery that Della, one of our favorite volunteers, had a moderately advanced case of TB shocked us. One lung was completely infiltrated, and her sputum showed TB organisms. It was a blow to this enthusiastic teenager to find that she was infectious and ill. Anxiously she sought information on how to take care of herself. Later in a home visit, both parents greeted the doctor, and there Della was, lying on her pallet.

They listened carefully to suggestions for their daughter's care. Della was to have complete bed rest except for trips to the toilet. She was to sleep downstairs away from the kitchen, and her folks would sleep upstairs until weather forced them down also. Her father promised to build Della a shelf for her own dishes and personal articles near her pallet.

Dr. Schwinge worried about keeping this active and intelligent young woman occupied. She suggested that Della make mukluks and have them sold through the store, after exposing them to the sun for several days to destroy any TB germs. Adelinda Womkon, who with Della had been interpreting for us, said Della was a good student. Adelinda was a bright girl of 16 or 18 who taught the primary grades, although she had received only an eighth-grade education.

Suddenly Dr. Schwinge thought of correspondence courses. Such a course would be ideal for Della if someone could write for her so that her papers would be clean. Adelinda immediately volunteered, saying that she would like very much to take a course herself and would be willing to work at some distance from Della; they both could learn together. Dr. Schwinge was so delighted she offered to pay for one course if they would study faithfully. Adelinda shyly told the doctor, "You have done much for us, and I have some money saved. I could pay for the course myself. It might be better for you to give your money to someone who did not have any." Dr. Schwinge was deeply touched. Later she told the story at dinner, saying, "By George, I like these Eskimos."

After I returned to Seattle around 1949 Adelinda came through with her church choir. I was honored that she looked me up and visited me. When I asked her what she would like to see, she pointed to the first thing on her list. It was the main Sears, Roebuck store. The young Eskimo woman, who had ordered from a Sears catalog all her life, was thrilled to walk through the store—to see and touch the merchandise instead of looking at pictures. The large store, with its rows and rows of appliances and apparel, impressed her far more than the skyscrapers, the crowds, or the Seattle traffic.

Dr. Schwinge and Kitty found our teaching materials were less and less effective. The films that had been so helpful in Southeast Alaska were no longer suitable. Kitty had to turn the script over to an Eskimo translator, who had problems keeping up because it took twice as long to say something in the Eskimo language as in English. She also was busy making a model of a room typical of this area, for a more effective teaching aid.

Toward the end of our stay, the villagers held a church service for the ship's personnel. The main attraction was the choir, which sang three songs. The small church was well filled. Soon it became very warm, but no one removed their parkas, not even the choir members, who sang with such gusto and volume that perspiration rolled down their faces. At the end of the service, Dr. Schwinge told the people how much we admired their village and their good spirit.

Then we moved outside for talk and to watch our crew meet the Natives' challenge for a tug-of-war. We didn't think the Eskimos had a chance of winning because they were so much smaller. Back and forth the two teams went, again with much shouting. The Eskimos soon demonstrated that the teamwork of their successive precise lunges would win over our crew's advantage in size. Later Eskimo women of all ages participated in a blanket toss, jumping to great heights and gracefully landing on their feet. None of us dared try it.

Kitty decided the Eskimos looked so young because the adults played right along with the children, enjoying games of muscular prowess as much as the little ones. We watched them dance. They did not have partners, but moved to the rhythm in one spot, telling their stories with expressive motions of their hands and bodies.

Mrs. Daugherty told us of an Eskimo woman, well advanced in years, who was going to church one Sunday morning carrying all the correct paraphernalia—Bible, hymn book, clean Sunday parka. She suddenly stopped, looked carefully around to make sure that no one was looking, and then quickly climbed the big "children's slide" (like those found in every schoolyard in the States) and slid down with an expression of joy on her face. She then calmly walked on to church.

As well as loving fun, the Eskimos were warm and appreciative of our efforts. Those who spoke English came up and said, "We like you, we hope you will come back again. Thank you for working so hard." The old women who could not speak English would come running up grinning, pounding their chests and waving their X-ray cards that were checked negative for TB saying, "Thank you, thank you," over and over again.

The town council expressed its gratitude to us when they gave Dr. Schwinge, Kitty, and me carved ivory dogs. Another woman gave each of us ink drawings done on walrus hide. The warmth and cheerful cooperation radiating from Gambell was in sharp contrast to its cold and surly surroundings. The world would be a more pleasant place if its so-called civilized people could learn some of the philosophy of living these Eskimos had developed. They cared and looked out for one another. They didn't strive to be first when there was a line-up, but rather they would say, "so-and-so is sick and needs it most." Mrs. Daugherty told us that to survive in this climate, the people had to cooperate and be able to depend on one another. An outstanding example of this caring love occurred when James brought some walrus meat aboard for Johnny Ivanoff. Johnny had been quite homesick for his own home diet, but had never mentioned the lack to anyone on the ship.

As we moved around the village, we saw that ivory carving was a popular occupation. We watched the carvers in fascination when we had the chance. One man operated a drill using both hands and his mouth. He supplied the power with his feet. Nearly every family had at least one person working on crafts. They were eager to sell or trade their works. Kitty and I each bought 22-piece carved ivory sets of all the birds, animals, and fish found on St. Lawrence Island. Our crew members were short of money, but they had developed their trading skills. We worried that they would not have any clothes left if the ship did not leave soon.

Toward the end of our stay the wind came up one morning and the skies cleared. We could see a faint outline of land on the distant horizon. This was Siberia, less than 50 miles away. Mrs. Daugherty explained that July used to be a time when many of the villagers would load their families into the skin boats and go across to visit with friends and relatives over there, or the Siberian Eskimos would come to Gambell. The Russians no longer allowed this.

In the six years the Daughertys taught at Gambell, they exerted a powerful influence on the culture of the town. Because the town had a generator and electricity, the school had a radio. Once a week Mr. Daugherty taught a news class. The students listened to a news broadcast. Then Mr. Daugherty explained in detail what had been said and filled in the background. This type of teaching certainly must have helped youngsters from such a remote village when they left to further their education later.

One evening we saw our old friend the *Square Knot* showing up on the horizon. Most of the people of the village had escorted us down to the beach. The older children insisted on carrying everything, including cameras and light meters. The adults could hardly wait to see what the *Square Knot* was bringing in the once-a-year shipment from the States.

We were low on fuel, and again the level in our water tanks was down to 200 gallons of rusty, lumpy, cider-colored fluid. After the freighter anchored, we tied up alongside to get fuel. Captain Steward, now on the final leg of his trip, pumped 2000 gallons of water into one of our cleaner tanks. Compared to the dirty stuff we had been drinking, this new water (still rationed) tasted like it had come from a sparkling mountain stream.

The surf was roaring up the beach again, and no umiaks came out to lighter the freight. Captain Steward was distressed at having to wait because he was far behind schedule. He told Dr. Schwinge he could only stay one more day, regardless of weather. "If the Eskimos don't get to work and unload the freight, they will have to wait until the *North Star* picks it up in

September and takes it to them." He explained that commercial ships had to be out of the Bering Sea by September 1, and that the canneries farther south were waiting for him. They were paying crews $15 a day to retain them for the necessary loading of the canned fish.

Dr. Schwinge understood how badly the village needed some of the equipment and supplies, so she passed the word to a village elder that if it was at all possible, he should try to get some men out to unload supplies. The next morning the umiaks were busily shuttling back and forth.

Part of the freight was a small caterpillar tractor. While they waited for the water to calm, the Eskimos fastened two of their largest skin boats together and built a platform on top large enough for the tractor. We watched, fascinated, as they towed the floating platform to the side of the freighter. There the crew members gently lowered the tractor onto the fragile structure. After the Eskimos secured the ungainly tractor, they carefully motored to a ramp they had built on the beach, where another tractor waited to pull it ashore. None of us could figure how the Eskimos managed to get the first cat ashore. By this time, however, we all recognized that the ingenious Eskimos could easily solve such a "weighty" problem.

Dr. Schwinge was worn out after dashing around and tying up loose ends before we left. She told us how she longed for her bed and a good night's sleep: she looked forward to clean sheets and pajamas after her weekly shower. The sea was calm, and she commented, "The *Hygiene* is certainly nice compared to the mobile health unit. I'm going to miss it when I leave." She started to crawl into her bunk, and discovered that it was completely soaked—two blankets, two clean sheets and one mattress.

At 1 a.m. no one was around as she fussed and fumed. This was the second time she had found her bed wet. Apparently the caulking in the deck seams over her bunk was faulty. She woke Mrs. Daugherty, Kitty and me for sympathy and to help her find a place to sleep. We found an extra mattress, put it on the floor, and covered her with our coats and jackets.

Gus and Wendell had their problems the next morning. The fuel they had obtained from the *Square Knot* had so much water in it that it would not burn. Gus had to drain 600 gallons of water off the 2000 gallons of "fuel" they had taken on from the freighter. Dr. Schwinge commiserated with him—"No hot food, no dry beds, I'm beginning to look forward again to the mobile unit!"

The next important strangers to step aboard would be Dr. Swanson, who would replace Dr. Schwinge, and a new secretary to take Mrs. Daugherty's place. We had expected them for several days, either by air or sea. Kitty and I hoped the replacements would be good shipmates and care about the villagers.

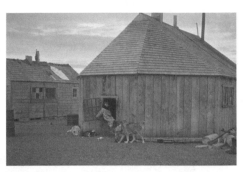

Top: eight-sided Siberian house.
Middle: left, child on beach;
right, Dr. Schwinge in Gamble.
Bottom: children playing
on beach at Gambell.

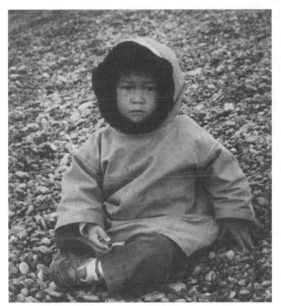

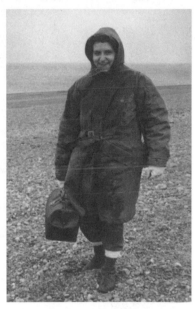

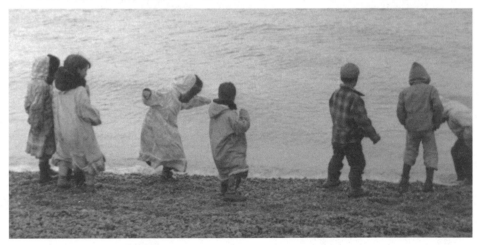

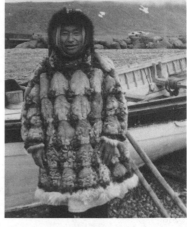

Top: Gambell man in feather parka.
Middle: left, Adelinda Womkon and older
woman celebrating TB negative;
right, Adelinda.
Bottom: Squareknot, unloading supplies.

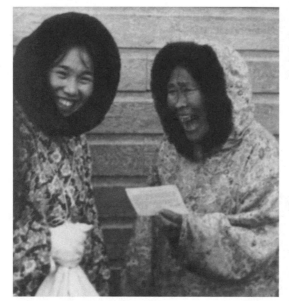

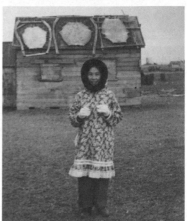

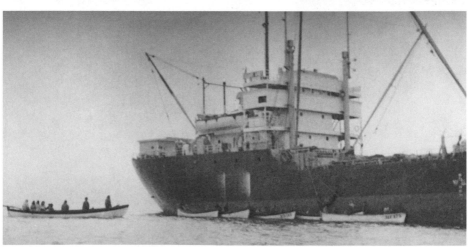

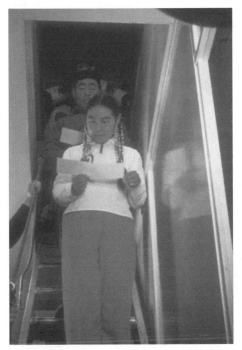

Left: top, Katherine Toolie;
middle, Savoonga.
Right: top, Katherine and
Eleanor in traditional
and modern fashions;
middle, Savoonga store.
Bottom: Savoonga beach.

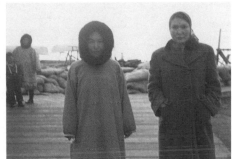

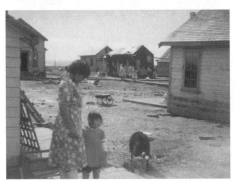

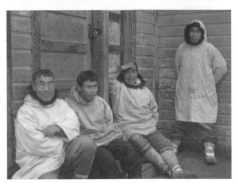

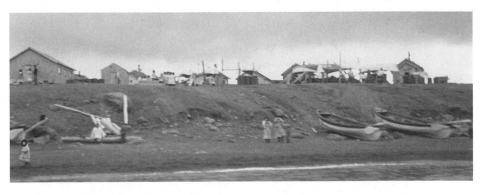

Savoonga
Tuesday, July 22, to Saturday, July 26

At last word came by radio on Monday, July 21, that Dr. Swanson and Miss MacNair, the new secretary, would arrive in Savoonga via Castell's mail boat on Tuesday. After a good night's sleep, the first in a long time, we left early Tuesday morning for the 50-mile trip eastward along the coast of St. Lawrence Island. It was slow going because only one of the *Hygiene's* engines was operating; the water in the fuel oil had put the other out of commission.

Sunshine and blue skies would have made our surroundings less forbidding, but everything was gray: the vast ocean, the threatening sky, and even the land lacked color. Except for one day, the weather had been almost constantly overcast.

Our tension built throughout the day. The difficulties with Dr. Krusich were still fresh in our memories, and we were not looking forward to working with an unknown quantity. Would Dr. Swanson understand the problems of weather and waves? Was he a good doctor? Would he stick with the present system, or would he want to change everything? We imagined and discussed all sorts of scenarios.

Dinner time came, and still no mail boat had appeared. We continued our incessant conversation about the new shipmates. The men of the crew were hoping for a beautiful young secretary. Kitty and I only wanted a dedicated, knowledgeable, good-natured, kind doctor with a sense of humor—in other words a clone of Dr. Schwinge. Conditions in the Bering Sea were far more demanding than elsewhere on our itinerary. Only a team working in full cooperation could accomplish the tremendous amount of work that had to be done during the short summer. We four medical staff members had been such a team, each one contributing respect, hard work, good humor, and sympathy for one another and for the Eskimos. The experience had been inspiring.

Dr. Schwinge, although young, had been a true leader and set the tone for the medical staff and the ship's crew. She and Captain Kippola had worked in harmony, and her sense of humor and fairness had helped the captain smooth over many of his problems with the crew. She was ambivalent about leaving in spite of the prospect of relief from the sea, which had no respect for her meals, her program, or her bed. When she first came aboard the *Hygiene*, she thought it would be a breeze compared to her truck unit where they had to find lodging and do their own cooking. But now, near the end of her stint on the *Hygiene,* she realized her decisions and responsibilities on the ship affected many more people than those she made on the truck unit. Though by now exhausted, she made it clear to us that she had enjoyed her tour on the *Hygiene* as much as her beloved truck.

In a letter to Dr. Albrecht, Dr. Schwinge later wrote, "I have a profound feeling of respect for every member of the crew and medical staff. The trip has been a grand adventure in God's beautiful world, and the camaraderie and friendships we have built are solid. The challenge of practicing medicine, the case-finding, and working with the wonderful people that we met were an experience I hope never to forget."

We hated to see Mrs. Daugherty leave. She had greatly enriched our understanding of the Eskimo, and had fit in competently wherever we needed her. Her sense of humor and consistent good nature made her a most valuable shipmate. We could not blame her for looking forward to getting back to her family and station at Golovnin.

About 8 p.m. Dr. Swanson and Peggy MacNair wearily climbed aboard the *Hygiene* from Castell's 45-foot mail launch. They would not soon forget the 140-mile trip from Nome. Sleeping bags on the open deck had been their only defense against the weather. All they wanted now was a warm place to sleep. Once we had made them comfortable, we became absorbed in our mail. Later, laughing, they claimed that it was the mail everyone wanted, not them. Again Dr. Pope was disappointed and angry because his instruments had not come.

Savoonga, a village of approximately 240 people, had a comparatively fine harbor and fresh water nearby. About 20 houses atop a small hill marked the townsite. Most of the buildings appeared to be one-room frame structures, with a few larger buildings scattered among them. Open spaces of wet ground crisscrossed by neat boardwalks separated the houses. The topography was entirely different from the barren gravel spit of Gambell, often referred to as the "city" of St. Lawrence Island because it was the destination for the larger boats and planes. Savoonga, a former reindeer-herding camp and an offshoot of Gambell, was the country town. Mrs. Daugherty indicated that the Savoonga craftsmen and people were not as skilled as those in Gambell.

The community store dominated the town and served as a gathering place for villagers, who sat warmly clothed on the stairs and eyed us curiously, although white men could not have been such an oddity, for many had visited the village. Maybe they found the white women a novelty.

On the whole, the interiors of the homes were clean and warm, a comfort after the cold outdoors. Dogs and drying walrus meat added to the atmosphere. The water supply came from a stream a quarter of a mile away. A neglected Caterpillar diesel furnished power for the light-plant, which barely put out sufficient voltage to run the projector. Kayak and umiak frameworks, some covered with skins, decorated the beach and hillside.

Savoonga was the best organized town we had ever visited. Mr. and Mrs. Williams, the school teachers, deserved the credit. Dr. Schwinge had told them that she and Dr. Swanson would like to start work at 9 a.m. Wednesday morning. Promptly at 8:30, a dory arrived at the *Hygiene* to take the two doctors ashore. It brought out volunteers with slips of paper giving their names and duties. The villagers came out in family groups with perfect timing. Each family was to get ready when their neighbors left for the boat. Men stationed on the beach expedited loading the umiaks. Even the weather cooperated. Between 9 a.m. and 4 p.m. Dr. Schwinge, with the help of the Willliamses and the interpreters, completed 128 physicals on the children. I took 223 X-rays, and Kitty drew 115 blood samples. The dentist extracted 32 teeth.

Dr. Schwinge introduced Dr. Swanson to our schedule and program, while Mrs. Daugherty explained the paperwork to Peggy, who proved to be beautiful, as the crew had requested, but not so young. She seemed intelligent, warm, and enthusiastic. The crew's consensus was, "She is a lady."

Dr. Swanson was of medium size and seemed well coordinated and energetic. He was rather quiet, though easy to talk to, and was probably a bit older than Dr. Schwinge. Peggy later told me a little about him. He was a native-born Alaskan from Valdez, had gone to Sheldon Jackson School in Sitka, earned his M.D. degree from the University of Chicago, and a master's degree in public health from Yale. His wife, in Juneau, was expecting their first child in three months.

In addition to Dr. Swanson and Peggy, the mail boat carried Dr. Thorne and a team from the Visual Aid Department of the Presbyterian Church of America. These men continued on to Gambell and planned to return to Savoonga the next day to photograph our work on the *Hygiene.*

They arrived about dinner time and rapidly transformed the clinic into a small bit of Hollywood. Spotlights and wires ran everywhere. A few villagers came out to work with us. The cameramen took stills and movies of all the procedures. At about midnight, Dr. Thorne and his photographers packed up their lights and cameras to load onto Castell's boat for the long, cold trip back to Nome. Dr. Swanson commented, "I don't envy them—yet. This has been quite a day for a starter."

We invited the Williamses and the Presbyterian lay worker for dinner on Thursday night. The men who sat next to the "missionary" complained that she had gone a little native, because she wore an odorous sealskin jacket and mukluks instead of cloth garments that could be laundered.

During dinner Mr. Williams told us stories about Mrs. Daugherty's earlier weekend visits, which sometimes ended up as three-week stays due to unexpectedly ferocious storms. Suddenly we felt the *Hygiene* begin to roll. While we were eating, the wind had changed to the northeast, and in a matter of minutes the harbor became untenable for the ship. Dr. Swanson, Dr. Pope, and Kitty had planned to go ashore after dinner to show movies, but now, traveling to shore was impossible for either staff or guests. As the rolling waves built in intensity, our company, one by one, lay down on the davenports in the dining salon. At first we teased them and laughed heartily. Then Dr. Schwinge started to get seasick, and she no longer thought it was so funny.

It was obvious that no one would return to shore that night. Unfortunately we did not have enough linens or bunks for our guests, but they did not care as long as they could lie down. Mr. Williams told the captain about a small, protected bay some three miles away. Immediately Captain Kippola gave orders to start the engines and weigh anchor. We scurried to gain shelter from the howling northeast wind. By morning the wind changed back to the east. The crew hauled up the anchor, and we prepared to move back to Savoonga, whose harbor was again protected.

While we maneuvered, the propeller cut the line securing the dory. Again we had a catastrophe—the wind blew our beautiful boat ashore, where the waves stove in its bottom against the rocks. Two of the men launched the little skiff and managed to get to shore and pull the dory up on the beach before it was completely ruined. It looked scary, as the seas were high and the skiff was out of sight half the time. Eventually we returned to Savoonga with our passengers and spent the rest of the day working on shore. The villagers welcomed us back as long-lost friends. Again they showed concern for our lack of local knowledge and the safety of their teachers.

While we worked in the village, the ship moved three miles to take on water from a small lake near the rocks where the dory had been smashed. In addition to helping the crew members with the water detail, the Eskimos patched the dory with impressive resourcefulness and skill.

Taking on water followed an ingenious procedure. First the men loaded buckets of water from the lake onto sleds that dogs pulled over the slippery dry grass to the top of the beach. There they poured it into a 50-gallon barrel. They then siphoned it down the hill into 50-gallon drums in the Eskimos' dories and ferried it to the *Hygiene,* where Gus pumped the water through a hose into the empty tanks. The Eskimos were exceedingly cooperative and worked with our crew most of one day and through the night. The *Hygiene* took on about 2500 gallons in this difficult manner.

An umiak ferried us from Savoonga back to the *Hygiene* when we finished our day's work. The Eskimos' seamanship impressed Dr. Swanson who, we learned, had spent some time working on a fishing boat. Kitty and I wanted to help with the water detail, but the most we could do was make sandwiches and feed the hungry gang in the middle of the night.

In the village, we saw results of our program everywhere. One father was out building two cupboards for the two patients with positive sputums in his home. In another home, the patient was asleep on her cot. The day before, she had been sitting on the floor in a corner. Dr. Schwinge's pink paper instructions on isolation procedures hung in all the homes in a conspicuous place.

As a whole, the St. Lawrence Island Eskimos seemed more receptive and eager for our services than any other group of people we had visited. Reports that the population of their island had a high incidence of TB had frightened them. Those who did not have the dreaded disease were doubly happy when they received their negative X-ray reports.

The 140-mile trip across the sea from the mainland had enabled the St. Lawrence Islanders to retain their original customs, houses, and clothes to a large extent. The distance, however, had not protected them from tuberculosis, which was as prevalent there as on the mainland.

We had completed a better and more generalized health program in Savoonga than in any other village we had visited in the Bering Sea, and there had been time to talk to and get to know the patients. The generally cooperative weather at this stop emphasized that bad weather was our greatest hazard to completing the program. Also the fresh water in our tank boosted our morale.

When we left on Saturday night, half the town was out on the beach to say good-bye. The girls who had helped wanted to come and work on the boat. Each Eskimo came up and shook every one of us by the hand. Many begged us to come back next year. Some of the women were crying as they said good-bye. We had lumps in our throats too.

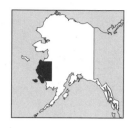

Yukon Delta

Nome to Mekoryuk
Sunday, July 27, to Thursday, July 31

We anchored about a mile off Nome after a delightful trip over calm seas. Dr. Schwinge, who had worked
on records until 2 a.m., threw her gear into a bag and
was ready, along with Mrs. Daugherty, to depart when the first shore boat
left. Both women knew all too well the fickleness of the weather, and they
were not taking any chances on being left aboard the *Hygiene*.

It was Sunday. Jessie and Ronald had the day off, so most of us spent the
entire day ashore exploring Nome. Dr. Swanson and Peggy felt like oldtimers,
having recently waited three days in the town for transportation to the
Hygiene. The community offered a hotel, a post office, a movie, three restaurants, several bars—and an ice-cream parlor.

Kitty and I visited Lois Morgan, the public health nurse, who lived in a
tiny, attractive house. There we learned at first hand about the sanitation
problems in the land of permafrost, where the ground never thaws more
than a few inches. The constant ice made it impossible to lay sewer pipes or
even dig holes for outhouses. People used "honey pots," the euphemistic
name for chemical toilets. Every few days the honey-pot man came around
to service the toilets of people who could afford to pay him. The fact that
many could not led to severe pollution problems, particularly in the Native
sections of the town.

Dr. Schwinge and Mrs. Daugherty shared a room at the hotel for $2.50
apiece. Dr. Schwinge paid $1.50 for a tomato and lettuce salad, and then
spent the afternoon sleeping. When she awakened, she invited us to use
the bathtub—oh, how grand to soak luxuriously in a tub full of hot water!
Mrs. Wallace, the hotel owner, took us on a tour of her greenhouse, where
it took all our willpower to keep from grabbing a handful of lettuce. We all
craved fresh vegetables after weeks of canned food.

The flat country around Nome with destinations several miles apart
was ideal for cyclers. Dr. Swanson and I rode the one and one-half miles to
see the King Islanders' summer village. Every year these Eskimos left
their craggy island and crossed nearly 100 miles of open water in their skin
boats to spend the summer in Nome. Once there, they turned the big umiaks upside-down on racks and hung canvas from the sides to form houses.
They sat there under their skin shelters, gossiping and chatting as they

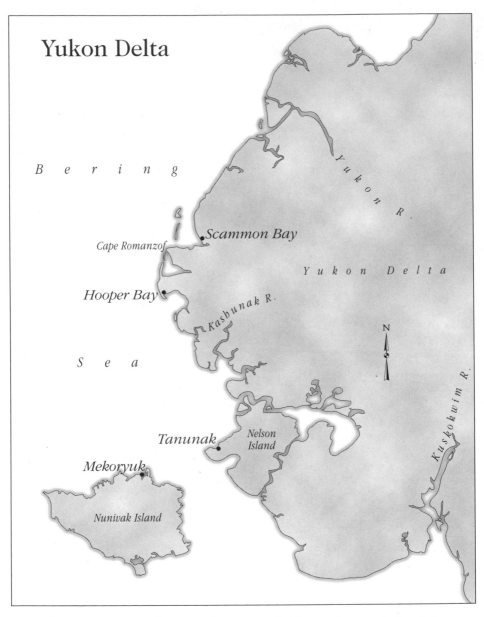

Yukon Delta

B e r i n g

Yukon R.

Scammon Bay

Cape Romanzof

Yukon Delta

Hooper Bay

Kasbunak R.

N

S e a

Kuskokwim R.

Tanunak

Nelson Island

Mekoryuk

Nunivak Island

This was the most difficult area for us to work. The weather was bad and the water so shallow that we could not even see the villages. One we never did find. The Natives had no concept of what we were trying to do and we had great difficulty communicating. In some ways they were more remote than the St. Lawrence Islanders in that it was much more difficult to reach their villages. The statistics on the low rate of venereal disease were evidence of this isolation.

carved ivory animals and cribbage boards and sold them to tourists. We biked on for two more miles to a fish camp, but it was so dirty and smelly we did not stay long.

Many of the Eskimos living on the outskirts of Nome apparently had lost both their self-respect and joy of living. They were so different from the happy, friendly people we had just left in Gambell and Savoonga. We wondered if the contrast between their life style and the white man's materialistic culture made them feel poor and insecure. Ready access to alcohol undoubtedly added to their problem. In the more remote villages, where the living conditions were similar for all, we noticed the people were busy with the mechanics of living and with helping their less fortunate neighbors.

That evening we went our separate ways. Dr. Swanson returned to the ship and moved into the doctor's stateroom, which had a few more conveniences than the fo'c'sle, the most notable being closet space. Dr. Schwinge and Mrs. Daugherty went to a movie. Johnny Ivanoff took Kitty and me for a ride in his brothers' car. We started to explore the hills behind Nome but soon turned back to escape the mosquitos.

When we returned to the ship, two of our shipmates were drunk. The first mate had quietly rolled into his bunk to sleep it off. Dr. Pope, on the other hand, repeatedly shot his gun into the air throughout his trip back to the ship from town. Even after he boarded the *Hygiene,* he continued his shooting spree. He was not rational, and it took both the captain and Dr. Swanson to forcibly take the gun from him. This episode frightened us all.

His wife tried to keep him in their small stateroom and had a hard time calming him down. They had married just before coming on board, and she had no idea of what she was getting into. The couple had pretty much kept to themselves and had consistently indicated they felt that they were just a little bit better than anyone else. Now, even though we would have liked to help her, Mrs. Pope did not feel she could confide in any of us.

On Monday Jessie went to town early and had a field day ordering groceries and meat, which, though not altogether fresh, were much better than anything she had had for a while. Dr. Swanson and Kitty were able to replenish some of the medical supplies. Then Dr. Swanson spent the rest of the day filling in at the busy Nome Medical Clinic because Dr. Tucker, the resident physician, was ill. The work consisted mostly of getting VD smears on female patients from the local jail. Miraculously, Peggy found someone to repair our ailing typewriter. After many delays, I was able to get a phone call through to my mother and was relieved to hear that all was going well.

Our dory busily ferried supplies and people back and forth all day. The dental instruments had not come, nor was there any mail. We all went ashore to bid goodbye to Dr. Schwinge and Mrs. Daugherty. They had been good friends, good shipmates, and an inspiration to us all. I was sad to see them leave and hoped our paths would cross again someday.

Toward the end of the day, the local Alaska Airlines station master sent word to Captain Kippola that a package for Dr. Pope had been shipped to St. Michael. That changed our planned arrival time at Akulurak, and Dr. Swanson sent a message notifying them we would be delayed in reaching the Yukon Delta.

Six-thirty a.m. found us anchored off St. Michael. We could not send the dory ashore because of a stiff east wind. About noon a plane arrived, and Captain Kippola made radio contact. He determined that no mail or dental instruments were there nor had any been delivered for the *Hygiene*.

In the clinic we kept busy with paperwork. Even Jessie was inundated with bookkeeping after her purchases in Nome. Whenever we had a busy work schedule, the paperwork mounded up in huge piles. We used every waiting period and calm travel time to catch up on recording.

At 2 p.m. Captain Kippola set a course for the Yukon Delta area, expecting to arrive in the early morning. A strong southwest gale blew up at midnight and made travel uncomfortable. We lay off the delta area until noon, but foul weather and only a half-mile of visibility in that shoal area did not encourage us to wait around for a good day. The captain and doctor decided to go on to Scammon Bay and attempt to find shelter behind Cape Romanzof.

That plan proved impractical. We could see the cape only occasionally in the distance through lifting clouds. The water was only four fathoms deep six to seven miles from shore. Anchoring closer to shore was impossible because of breakers. The next choice was to buck on down to the nearest shelter, Nunivak Island, and work there as long as the weather was bad.

We anchored in the shelter of Cape Etolin, Nunivak Island, at 3 a.m. The ship stopped its violent rolling and pitching, and after a few hours of greatly needed and appreciated peaceful sleep, we inspected the clinic. The ship had taken such a severe pounding that the deck seams had opened and salt water had leaked over everything in the clinic. The floor was awash and water had dripped over the X-ray transformer and short-circuited the dryer-fan line. Gus came to the rescue and rewired a different fan into the X-ray film drier. Mopping up and checking the equipment occupied most of the day. By late afternoon everything seemed to be back in order, and we rounded Cape Etolin to try and find Mekoryuk.

Visibility was poor, and we were directly off the village before we could distinguish it about two miles distant. The southwest wind prevailed, but the captain found a lee inside a reef a mile or more out from the village.

Mekoryuk
Thursday, July 31, to Monday, August 4

After dinner Dr. Swanson, Kitty, and I put in to shore with several Eskimos who came out in a rowboat to investigate us. Wearing life jackets, we rode the surf into a small protected bay in front of the village. Later, Gus told us that the little boat bobbed up and down so much in the waves, we had been out of sight most of the time. From shore, Dr. Swanson set up radio contact with Captain Kippola and informed him of a more protected anchorage, to which he immediately moved.

We returned to the ship at its new location at 11 p.m. in total darkness. The new route entailed crossing a bay in the Eskimos' skiff. The bay was so shallow that when the tide was out, as it was, the men climbed out and shoved their boat, with us in it, through the mud, squishing with each step. Next we hiked across a quarter-mile of tundra. The teachers and Eskimos had warned us to be wary of the musk ox that roamed the area. The government was trying to establish a herd on the island. The beasts were large and purported to be vicious. No one advised what we should do if we met one of them in the dark.

When we saw the lights of the *Hygiene* in the distance and heard the welcome sound of John's halloo as we approached the beach, we relaxed a bit. Midnight found us safely on the *Hygiene*. We figured if we could survive the trip in total darkness, it should be passable for the village people in daylight.

We had arrived two weeks earlier than the teachers, Mr. and Mrs. Herman Turner, had expected. The storm had literally blown the *Hygiene* past the intervening stops. It was unfortunate that we had arrived unexpectedly in this remote traditional village. However, everyone set to and made the best of it.

The next morning interpreters and ushers arrived with a large group of women and children. To Kitty and me, it was the usual jam session of crying youngsters and confused adults. Dr. Swanson and Peggy, who had seen only the very well-organized and well-behaved people of Savoonga, described the session as bedlam. Peggy had the usual difficulty in keeping the family records straight, due to the various adoptions, stepchildren, and changes in family names. Some of the children were listed under three different family names.

The interpreters and ushers did not understand what they were to do and wandered off to explore the ship. The pace of our work slowed to a crawl, since we were totally dependent on the interpreters.

When I began X-raying, I discovered that several contact points on the voltage regulator of the X-ray machine had corroded when the salt water sprayed the clinic. I could not make the adjustments necessary to take good X-rays. A line of confused Eskimos waited while Gus and Dr. Pope quickly devised new brushes for the regulator. It was impossible to explain the delay to these people who knew nothing about electricity or X-rays. Their language had no words to fit the situation. I held my breath and prayed with each X-ray that the whole tube would not blow. It held together until midnight, when I took the last X-ray for that day.

None of the patients scheduled for follow-up X-rays arrived on the following morning. In fact, no one arrived. Again our outboard was not functioning, due this time to a broken propeller. Resignedly, John rowed ashore to find out what was causing the delay. Donald Baker, an excellent interpreter and intermediary, explained that the *Hygiene's* anchorage, ideal in a southwest wind, was now less than desirable after the wind slackened. The captain and doctor decided to move the ship around to anchor one and a half miles off shore in front of the village. Kitty, Peggy and I seized the opportunity to catch up on record work. After the move we were able to continue our program.

Some interesting statistics showed up in our records. Mekoryuk had very few people over the age of 60 and practically no children between the ages of six and 10. Questioning revealed that in the early 1940s, a measles outbreak had taken its toll of infants and older people. The Turners told us that about every other year large numbers of babies were born. This was an off-year, with only three pregnancies. The mothers in this village nursed their children for two to three years and carried the youngsters around on their backs, in some instances up to the age of five or six years. By that time some of the children looked as if they should be carrying the mothers.

The children cried very readily, perhaps because of the ordeal of divesting them of parkas and three to four layers of clothing underneath. The tiniest of infants was dressed from head to toe in much the same manner. All the clothing and crying made it imperative that the parents undress the children in another room so the examiner and the unclothed children being examined could be out of earshot of the rioting.

Kitty tried to stimulate the women's interest in better prenatal and delivery care. The town did not even have a midwife box with equipment essential to safe birthing. She also tried to promote the idea that town councils could sponsor beds in the TB sanitariums, thereby providing more funds for isolating and caring for their own TB patients. Many of the towns had community funds for various purposes, such as recreation, and gas for dories to come to the *Hygiene,* projects they could see, but sponsoring a bed in an unknown sanitarium was a difficult concept for them to grasp.

Mekoryuk was by far the least developed village we had seen. Most of these people lived in barabaras—10- by 12-foot holes in the ground covered with sod roofs. The only light source was a sealskin skylight, and the entry a tunnel. Five to ten people might live in each shelter. Donald Baker explained, "The houses are warm, but you would not like the smell."

Large cooking pots hung over open fires outdoors. When the hunters caught fish or birds, they dropped them whole into the cauldrons, and when the members of the family became hungry they fished something out. Rotting reindeer carcasses and drying fish littered the ground. Hungry sled dogs roamed everywhere, quarreling over the offal.

The local water supply came from various sources—pools about the filth-strewn barabaras and from a spring a mile up the river. The Turners were constructing a well about 50 feet behind the schoolhouse. They boiled all the water used at the schoolhouse, but no other homes followed that procedure.

In the summer the populations of two communities crowded the area when the people of Nash Harbor joined their Mekoryuk neighbors to work at the reindeer plant. Mr. McClellan of the Alaska Reindeer Service took us on a tour of his butchering facility, capable of handling 5000 deer. He showed us the corrals, butchering area, and refrigeration plants to the west of the village. They were trying to keep the reindeer population low enough so that overgrazing would not endanger the feeding grounds. The plant made hamburger of the hindquarters of adult reindeer and sent it to all the Native institutions. They gave the forequarters and necks to the Eskimos for their own use.

The Eskimos cached their personal meat supplies about the corrals and grounds. Putrefaction would set in before the plant operators found and disposed of these aging carcasses. This caused some antagonism among the Eskimos. A few villagers dissected the meat and dried it for winter feed. The air of the community reeked of spoiling meat and fish, which dried very poorly in the damp, cold air.

All these facilities were fenced in; entry was through a turnstile. McClellan explained the difficulties of the operation—the Eskimos worked enthusiastically until the first paycheck. Then, with money in their pockets, they could see no need for working again until it was gone. They delighted in butchering, bloodshed, and skinning, but it was difficult to get them to clean up the gore and mess. This task was delegated to boys aged 15 to 20, whose great pleasure was hosing each other down while neglecting the corners of the sheds.

Mrs. Schaubel, the ANS nurse from Bethel, flew in to join us while we worked in her territory. We found this gray-haired, older, no-nonsense nurse a great help to us, because she knew "her people." She explained that this was a summer village and not typical of where the families spent the greater part of the year. Dr. Albrecht had sent a letter to Dr. Swanson requesting that the *Hygiene* work the Kuskokwim area, since many of the Natives were now located along the banks of the river in their fishing camps. After a general staff meeting, the captain and doctor decided that because we only had a month left of "good" weather and were already behind schedule, we had better not add to the itinerary. Mrs. Schaubel, familiar with the area, agreed, saying moorage in the river at Kuskokwim could be difficult for the *Hygiene*.

On Sunday morning the sun was warm and the wind calm. Dr. Swanson came in for breakfast and surprised us when he said, "You know, in spite of all our difficulties, the work here is essentially finished. Let's take the day off and enjoy our surroundings." Only the Popes, focused on getting home, dissented.

When Donald Baker found out that we were not working that day, he invited Dr. Swanson, Kitty, Johnny Ivanoff, and me to go for a ride up the river in his outboard. In five minutes I threw together a picnic lunch of cans of baked beans, crushed pineapple, and a loaf of bread.

After we passed through the town, a reindeer swam across the river and gave us an excellent opportunity to take close-up pictures. We searched the shores for the formidable musk ox. For the first time in weeks, it was comfortably warm outdoors. What joy! At lunch time Donald pulled the boat onto a flower-covered bank, where we ate our peculiar lunch.

Then we lay on the colorful carpet of flowers absorbing the bird songs, the fragrance, and the peace of being away from the constant hum of the ship's motors. Later we strolled through the fields of wildflowers, all the time keeping one eye peeled for the ferocious musk ox. Only the litter of broken reindeer horns gave evidence of the large population of animals. I took a perfect set of horns back to the ship as a souvenir. Del quickly mounted them atop the *Hygiene's* mast.

When we returned to the village, I wandered along the beach looking at the kayaks pulled up on the shore. They were roomier than my baidarka, shorter and with a single cockpit. I was eager to try one but could not make anyone understand what I wanted until Johnny came by. After a long conversation with a couple of men he said, "They don't think you can do it by yourself. But I'll borrow two so I can go with you. I don't know any more about paddling than you do, but it will be fun, and they will feel better." When the people of the village heard that a white lady was going to try to paddle one of their kayaks, many came down to watch the fun.

These Eskimos did not know that their kayaks were much wider, more comfortable, and considerably less tippy than the baidarka. I could sit on the bottom and put my feet out in front of me, thus obtaining far more stability than was possible in the kneeling position. Although I could not understand the words, the Eskimo's gestures made it evident that they were sure I was going to tip over in the cold water.

When they pushed us off the beach I gave a little wiggle to see how tippy the boat felt. Suddenly the voices on shore were silent. That was when I was supposed to capsize. The crowd on the beach seemed disappointed when I paddled off with no problems. Again I fell in love with a boat.

After that short paddle, I knew I had to have a real Eskimo kayak. When we landed, Johnny wandered along the beach with me to see if we could find one for sale. At last he found a man who showed some interest.

After talking to him, Johnny asked me, "Would you be willing to offer him $80?"

Quickly I nodded, "Yes."

Johnny explained, "They don't have any wood to make a new framework. Driftwood is scarce around here, and the bushes are too small to provide branches, but if you pay him enough he will part with it."

I asked, "Would it be right to take away something he can't replace?"

Johnny explained my worry to the owner of the kayak. He smiled, nodded his head and handed me the paddle. Johnny said that the fellow was hoping to get enough money for a skiff and an outboard motor. The village was in transition from watercraft of the Native culture to modern boats and gasoline engines.

The others returned to the ship in the outboard, while I proudly paddled out in my new-found treasure, thinking how comfortable and stable it was, and hoping I would have time to use it. I had warned the former owner that if Captain Kippola said "No" to my purchase, I would have to bring it back. With a little persuasion I convinced the captain that this kayak was much safer than the baidarka, which I would sell at the first opportunity. He gave me permission to stow one more boat on the upper deck.

All had not been well on the ship while we were away. Ronald, walking past the clinic door, had smelled smoke and found it billowing up from the clinic's lower deck. A fire, the most feared disaster at sea, was burning somewhere below. He called Gus, who traced the smoke to a short-circuited wire below the X-ray equipment on the port side, behind the new water tank—a most difficult place to reach. Gus crawled through the bilges with a fire extinguisher to squelch the flames and was almost overcome by smoke. Kitty was concerned about Gus and the smoke he had inhaled. Frightened, we all wondered when, where, and if another short might occur. We spent the rest of the evening checking electrical connections, and cleaning the clinic.

The many positive X-rays showed that the town was a hotbed of TB. Tremendous crowding, poor air circulation, and lack of medical understanding made the situation seem hopeless. Kitty suggested that the town apply for a government housing loan, as Hoonah had done in Southeast Alaska.

Dr. Pope commented that the village people, in contrast to the TB situation, had the most perfect teeth he had seen.

Mekoryuk was an outstanding example of the importance of preparing the town and teachers for the *Hygiene's* services. Our schedule did not allow for preparation after our arrival. Even if the teachers knew we were coming, which only happened about half the time, a late telegram could not adequately communicate the high degree of cooperation required from the villages if we were to complete our work. We hurried into a town expecting to be operating in full swing within an hour. But the Eskimos lived at a much slower pace, and our time meant nothing to them. Teachers were the necessary connecting link to motivate villagers, but with no prior warning even the best teacher could not herd people several miles over land and water to the ship in an hour's time.

We hoped in the future the health department could prepare the villages by letter, in addition to notification by radio. We had to remind ourselves constantly that this was a program in the experimental stage, and we could not expect perfection the first time around.

Scammon Bay, Hooper Bay, and Kashunak
Tuesday, August 5, to Tuesday, August 12

When we left Mekoryuk, I thought we had probably seen everything the Bering Sea could throw at us, both good and bad. We all hoped the going would be easier for the next month. But more trouble was to come.

Captain Kippola backtracked and again searched for Scammon Bay. Through the morning he zigzagged back and forth parallel to the shore, looking for a channel. Twice we grounded on the bottom 20 miles out from the invisible

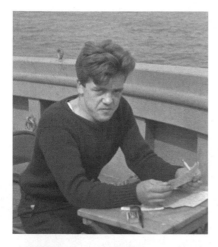

Top: Dr. Swanson.
Middle: left, Nome ;
right, Dr. Schwinge in Nome.
Bottom: King Island umiak at Nome.

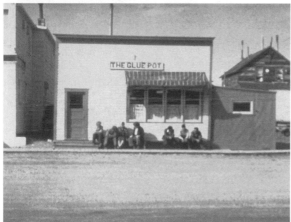

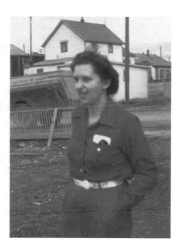

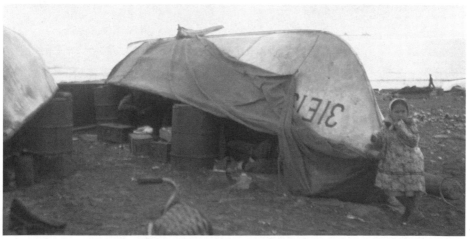

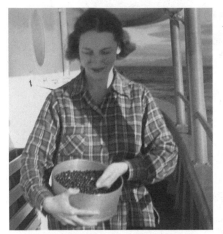
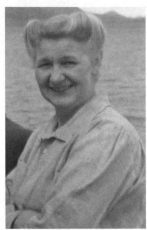

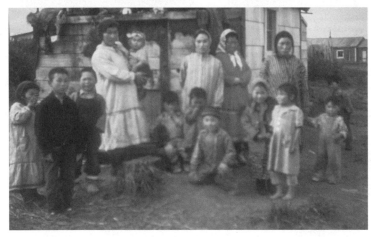

Top: left,
Peggy;
right, Mrs.
Schaubel.
Middle: family
in front of
their house,
Mekoryuk.
Bottom:
barabara at
Mekoryuk.

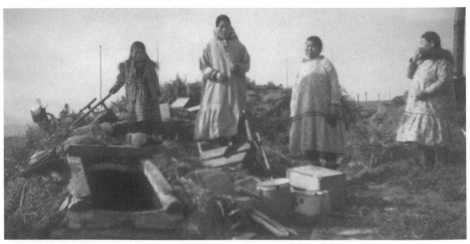

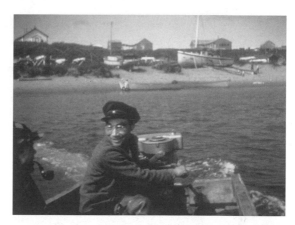

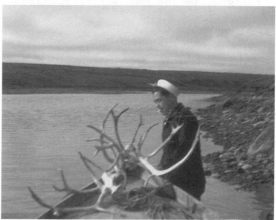

Top: Donald Baker at Mekoryuk.
Middle: Johnny and the reindeer horns we collected.
Bottom: reindeer factory at Mekoryuk.

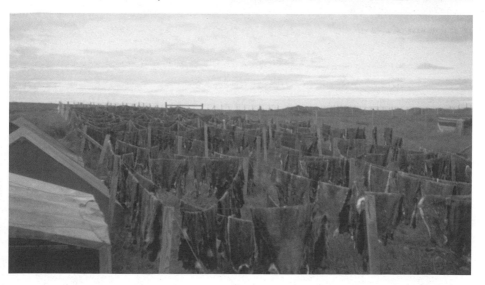

village. After backing off both times with no damage, the captain decided not to press his luck, and he headed for Hooper Bay.

There he found an anchorage near shore, about four miles from the barely visible town. We waited, hoping that someone would come out to the ship. When no one appeared, Dr. Swanson, Kitty, Mrs. Schaubel, and Johnny Ivanoff rowed ashore and started walking toward the village. From this point on, confusion reigned. Fortunately two Eskimos working at a reindeer camp down the beach saw the strangers and came running to talk to them. The Eskimos explained that they were on a peninsula and were indeed headed for Hooper Bay, but in order to cross to the town, they had to head in the opposite direction for a mile in order to reach a ford across the slough that separated the town from the peninsula. The men took them back to the river and then up the stream to the village in their dory. After hiking another half mile, the shore party reached the schoolhouse. By then it was 4 p.m.

Most of the time at Hooper Bay remains a blurred confusion in my mind, but a few vignettes stand out sharply. One day while I was on deck looking for a boatload of patients, I saw an Eskimo paddling a one-hole kayak past the *Hygiene.* His wife was sitting behind him facing the back of the boat. On the deck in front of her were three children graduating down in size, each holding the one in front of him. Two more children sat in front of the paddler. The kayak was nearly under water. Kayaks certainly were the most practical boat for getting about in that area.

Sandbars were everywhere. Almost every night the group riding in our dory had to get out and shove it through the mud. The area seemed like a giant sponge, with no rhyme or reason to its shoreline and channels.

Camille, a young man from Kashunak, and a teen-age boy and girl acted as interpreters and helped me with the X-rays. They were very smart and learned so quickly that I thought the boy could have been taking X-rays in another day. He would have liked to work on the boat permanently, and I would have liked to have him. These local youngsters helped us immensely. In addition, we hoped it would also encourage and inspire them to go to school for further training so they could come back to help their people.

Kitty raved about Mildred Jacobsen, a young Eskimo woman with a high-school education. The mother of five children, she was expecting another shortly. With a local woman aide, she taught about 45 students. The school was immaculate, with varnished desks, oiled floors, and white starched curtains at the windows. Kitty thought Mildred was one of the most remarkable teachers she had met.

One night when the rest of the medical staff was ashore, Mrs. Pope, Ronald, Del, and I were preparing the X-ray cards, normally a rather boring job. Suddenly Ronald burst out laughing, "Listen to this," he chortled as he wrote a name on the card, "Pop Eye," then "Andy Gump." Soon Mrs. Pope came across "Abe Lincoln." We discovered the Fishes, the Browns, the Greens, O'Briens, and David Bunyan all mixed in with the Tomangunaks, Nayaraks, and Ayagaraks. Later Father Convert, the Catholic priest who had lived there 15 years and was translating the Bible into Upik, told us that a long time ago, one of the Catholic missionaries had persuaded some of the Eskimos to give up their Upik names and adopt English ones. Some of them had done so, using odd sources.

I remember the confusion and pressure of X-raying 250 patients from two villages. We had to complete all the work on those who had come 20 miles by small boat early enough for them to return the same day. There was no place for them to stay in Hooper Bay. Over 50 positive cases entailed so much lab work I was only able to leave the ship once while we were there. My only recollections of the town were about 50 barabaras that seemed larger than those at Mekoryuk.

Kitty, Dr. Swanson, and Mrs. Schaubel spent every day and most evenings in the village holding clinics and demonstrating and teaching isolation techniques. In some cases TB had infected every member of the family.

Mrs. Schaubel spent one night with Mildred and her children in order to wash some of our bed linens and to escape the constant rolling of the ship. Again we had no clean linens left. Her one night ashore turned into two when the wind came up; again no one could go out in the small boats.

Father O'Connor, the village priest, told Dr. Swanson that nine infants younger than one year had died the previous winter of unknown causes. Some families had only one living child, although the mothers had borne innumerable babies. Dr. Swanson commented that here again, the mothers nursed the children for two to three years on average and carried them about until they were three or four. He decided this latter peculiarity was not such a bad idea, when he considered the nomadic nature of the people. They moved seasonally from fish to reindeer camps. The boggy tundra made walking difficult, even for adults, and the unstable mounds of moss and tall grass hummocks in swampy areas were completely impassable for small children during the spring, summer, and fall months.

Dr. Swanson reported many patients suffering from heart murmurs, rheumatic pains, and follicular tonsillitis, the result of former strep infections. He also observed many eye problems and cases of blindness.

It wasn't surprising that colds were going around the ship. Those who went ashore often missed dinner and didn't return until 11 or 12 p.m., usually soaking wet from wading through the mud. They had to be up and ready for work at 8 a.m. in case the boats arrived with patients. Dr. Swanson started giving vitamins to the crew and staff as well as to patients.

At last our stay was over, and the *Hygiene* wormed her way out of the bay through the sandbars. Captain Kippola proceeded slowly and with great care until we were 20 miles from shore. Even then, we encountered unexpected sandbars.

Aboard ship for the first time in weeks, we had a chance to sit around the table and talk to one another. The magnitude of managing the TB problem was so great that no simple answer was apparent. Hospitalizing active TB cases in order to stop the cycle of infection seemed to be the best solution. But the hospitals were so distant, not only in miles but also in culture and language, that in many cases a nearly total breakup of family life would result.

Kitty and I reminisced about our first few months aboard the *Hygiene* in Southeast Alaska: how we had worried about the stark living conditions (unpainted houses had seemed "primitive" then); how the Natives had to travel 40 or 50 miles, not hundreds, to get to a doctor or a hospital; how in fact a few of the older people could not understand English; how we sometimes had to anchor out in front of a village instead of docking.

Then we remembered crossing the Gulf of Alaska, running into storms and having to anchor in unprotected situations—but even then we could nearly always find shelter. Never until now had we been where the sea was so constantly rough, where the anchorages were so poor, the amenities of living conditions so minimal, language differences so great, and the need for medical help so overwhelming. We realized that all of these factors contributed to the difficulty of working in the area and emphasized the need for continuous and concentrated health service.

On the positive side, Dr. Swanson pointed out the low rate of venereal disease (no doubt due to the villages' isolation and extremely difficult access), and Dr. Pope added that in spite of the people's limited diet, he had seen fewer dental caries here than anywhere in his experience. That brought up the need for nutrition education, especially on using indigenous foods and preparing them for winter storage. We needed posters and movies that the Eskimos could understand.

Peggy, who had been listening quietly, commented that she had never seen so much record work that had to be done under such difficult conditions. A town of about 300 people generated 1600 records. Two or three of us wrote steadily for three to four hours to accomplish this task at each village. Peggy had had trouble adjusting to our extremely long and irregular hours.

Tanunak
Tuesday, August 12, to Saturday, August 16

After an uneventful trip we anchored five miles out from the village of Tanunak. It was barely visible through the dusk and mist. Dr. Swanson, Kitty, Peggy, Wendell, Ronald, Del, and John all loaded into the dory and headed into the village. Sometimes the crew members, whose duties kept them on board most of the time, thought that the trips ashore to make contacts were a lark, and they wanted to go along. They learned otherwise this time. Peggy reported that on the way in, they ran over several sandbars and had to stop the motor and row until they found deeper water. On reaching shore, they waded 50 feet through knee-deep mud, dragging the dory behind them.

Mr. and Mrs. Clifton Meyer, Tanunak's young and energetic teachers, greeted them on the beach. They warned that the tide was going out, so the sightseers made a quick tour of the town. Kitty, and Dr. Swanson obtained the village census, explained the program, and made arrangements for the next day. Twenty-six minutes after they had landed, the group returned to find the dory high and dry on the sand. The seven of them tugged and dragged it, wading through the mud and water for a mile before they floated and could start the motor. John said it was lucky he had the extra help. Peggy decided she would choose her shore expeditions more carefully.

Back at the ship the doctor, Kitty, and Peggy worked on the census and filled out forms until 1 a.m. to prepare for the crowd the next morning. I had succumbed to the shipboard cold going around and went to bed before the others returned. Dr. Swanson wrote in his journal: "Quite a day. With all the rowing and hauling a person has to do in this Bering Sea country, I feel as though I were back on a fishing boat."

When Dr. Swanson and Mrs. Schaubel went ashore in the forenoon to hold clinics, they found that the Eskimos were making no effort to leave for the *Hygiene*, although the water was reasonably calm and the tide right. Dr. Swanson had to ask the priest, Father Deschaut, and Mr. Meyer to tell the people of the village to get out to the ship immediately if they wanted medical attention.

Father Deschaut, who was from Belgium, had lived in the village 14 years and spoke the Yupik language fluently. He understood the Eskimos' lack of concern about time and was a great help in persuading them we would not wait around. Soon a steady stream of boats ferried patients back and forth whenever the tide permitted. By Wednesday night I had finished most of the X-raying. The work went smoothly because many of the people spoke English.

Johnny Ivanoff became sick with pharyngitis and was running a fever. The doctor told him to stay in bed in the fo'c'sle. Some of the crew members grumbled that he was being babied; no one else had been put to bed with their colds.

I caught up with my work and got a ride to the town at the end of our stay. On my way to the store, I noticed a few barabaras, but most of the homes were of frame construction. The store had a good selection of mats, rugs, and baskets woven from the native grasses, in addition to the usual canned goods, cigarettes, candy, and soft drinks. I could not resist buying some of the baskets and a couple of rugs, even though I wasn't sure where I could put them.

Just as I was leaving the store, I spotted a pair of very long lightweight mukluks far back in a corner. "May I try them on?" I asked one of the boys.

"Sure," he replied, "They are water mukluks and will keep your feet and legs dry. We need 'em in the mud-flats around here."

They proved to be just what I needed for getting in and out of my new kayak. Made of seal gut and fastened securely with broad straps tied around the ankle as well as below and above the knee, they would not pull off when I walked in the mud. They fit perfectly. I bought them for $7.50.

Thinking it would be fun to wear my new mukluks while visiting the schoolteachers, where I was to meet Kitty, I put them on and grandly made my appearance, only to have Kitty rapidly usher me outdoors until I had removed them. Still recovering from a cold, I had lost my sense of smell. "The mukluks," Mr. Meyers explained, "are tanned in urine and are extremely foul smelling."

When Mr. Meyers found out that I had a kayak and liked to paddle, he borrowed one for me. I had not paddled mine in from the *Hygiene* because the distance was too great for safety. In fact, I had not had any opportunity to paddle my new kayak. While Kitty was showing movies in the schoolhouse, I paddled up the gently moving stream that ran behind the town. After negotiating a few bends, I left behind all signs of civilization. Each curve brought a new vista as I slid quietly along the edge of the stream, sneaking close to feeding birds, who ignored my presence. Wildflowers covered the banks in a profusion of colors. A fragrant wind blowing through the grasses was also bringing more and more clouds. The pleasure of pushing the paddle in the water and feeling the response of the silent kayak urged me to keep going. But the wind was steadily increasing, and I knew the others would worry about me. Reluctantly I headed back.

Out on the bay, a severe storm had come up. The Eskimos had moved their boats to a slough behind the village to protect them from the pounding waves. They could not move them out until the next high tide occurred and the wind died.

Meanwhile Captain Kippola, unable to make radio contact with shore, sat on the *Hygiene* worrying about what had happened to us, and what was going to happen to the *Hygiene*, as he was more or less obligated to remain where he was until he could contact us. The captain had developed an understandable phobia about using the ship's dory, so he would not lower it. Meanwhile we waited for him to send it in to pick us up. The intensity of the storm kept increasing. By 7 p.m. it was obvious that we could not return to the ship. The Meyerses took us in, and we had a delightful evening with them and Father Deschaut. We discovered Dr. Swanson's flexible and happy personality when he was not under the pressure of work. He laughed as he said, "We're marooned; let's enjoy ourselves. We have good company, food, and a place to sleep, thanks to the Meyerses, and it isn't rolling. It's up to the captain to send a boat in for us."

They told us about the people in the village. The Hoopers were Tanunak's most prominent citizens. Twenty-nine-year-old George, the oldest son, had suffered a birth deformity of both legs; when he stood up, they flexed backward at the knees by 70 degrees. Therefore, he walked on his knees, protected by leather pads, with a fast, waddling gait. George had an amazing sense of balance and could get in and out of small boats better than many men with normal legs. He ran the store, waited on people, and was the best hunter and trapper in the village. Alexander, the middle brother, who had the same affliction, was also very adept. Much credit could be given to their parents who faithfully and patiently taught the boys to get along in the world.

The youngest boy, age 12, had been sent to Children's Orthopedic Hospital in Seattle for corrective surgery to straighten his legs. They now looked normal, but the operation left him weak and fearful, still dependent on crutches. The soft, muddy ground and slippery boardwalks made it difficult for him to move around, whereas his brothers walked confidently on their padded knees. The older boys were strong, agile, confident, and jolly young men. We reflected that maybe modern medicine didn't have all the answers.

After a good dinner provided by the Meyerses, and an evening of stimulating conversation, we turned in on assorted pads and beds with the wind howling in our ears. We wondered how the others were making out aboard the *Hygiene*.

The wind had subsided a bit the next morning, but the Eskimos did not want to move any boats from the protection of the slough. When no boat appeared from the *Hygiene,* and Mr. Meyers was unable to contact Captain Kippola on the radio, he suggested a trip across the slough to the site of an ancient community. Happily we loaded into two small boats and crossed the protected stream behind the village. With picks and shovels, we took off across the tundra, each of us certain that he would make the archeological find of the century. At the site of the historical village, we dug and rummaged around in the gravel for about an hour. I found a smooth rock that looked as though someone might have painted a sun with rays on it. We failed to unearth anything else of interest.

The men shot five geese, and we women picked a large can of berries and a bag of greens. About 2 p.m. we headed back to Tanunak to feast on our harvest. When we reached the village the *Hygiene's* dory was approaching from the ocean. Dr. Pope and Wendell, in life jackets, were coming for us. Unfortunately, when the wind died enough for the two men to lower the dory, the tide had started to fall, and thus two more were added to the group stranded ashore. The bay was a sea of mud, and it would be impossible to leave before the early evening tide came in.

Dr. Pope reported that the captain was in a fury. He could not understand what had kept us ashore, and he was taking his anger out on those left aboard. Wendell said the previous night was the roughest he had spent on the ship. The crew was ready to walk off at the first available port.

We returned to the ship rested and relaxed, only to find anger and depression. The captain had totally alienated the crew. I was afraid he was close to a nervous breakdown.

Dr. Swanson now was sure that Johnny had rheumatic fever and should be hospitalized. He was running a high fever and had painfully swollen ankle and knee joints. Rolling around in his bunk on the ship was hardly the best treatment for him. The already overworked and angry crew refused to pitch in and help with his work. As a result, the captain was standing his watches alone.

It had been a long hard summer, especially for Captain Kippola. He had guided a ship not designed for Bering Sea conditions through consistently rough water, and had anchored in dangerously shallow, exposed sites in his attempts to make the *Hygiene* accessible to the Eskimos.

I understood the crew's anger at Captain Kippola, but I worried about our safety, with only one exhausted man on the bridge for six hours at a time. I made it a point to be on the bridge when he was on watch. He was so grateful for company that he did everything he could to keep me entertained. We talked about one of my dreams of being a licensed seaman and working my way up to being a mate. He didn't think that was practical, as most ships didn't have quarters for women. He taught me many tricks of seamanship and let me plot courses. While I relieved him at the wheel, he told me endless stories of the sea and read poetry of all kinds. I found him fascinating when he relaxed a bit.

He worried excessively about many things, some of which he had no control over: for instance, the beating the *Hygiene* was taking, the rough weather, the tight schedule, the dory problems, and the crew's attitude. An immediate problem was cleaning the clinic. The crew had flatly refused to work except their twice-a-day six-hour shifts, and with Johnny assigned to bed rest, no one was available to scrub the clinic and clean the heads. In his hours off, the captain was doing Johnny's work. Kitty and I tried to help, but most of the time we were already putting in 16-hour days and had neither time nor energy to do more.

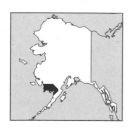

Bristol Bay Area

Goodnews Bay, Platinum, and Mumtrack
Sunday, August 17, to Monday, August 25

In the afternoon, a short distance out of Platinum, we felt some bumps and a solid thump. The *Hygiene* had run hard aground. The charts showed plenty of water for our position, but we were stuck fast. The rising wind gave the ship such a hard pounding that Gus was afraid the rudder post might break loose. Fortunately, a shallow-draft power barge out of Platinum came alongside and pulled us off the bar into a deep channel.

A short time later the anchor went over the side in the protected waters of Goodnews Bay. The rudder post had held, and tantalizing odors drifted out from the galley. Kitty was cooking a Sunday dinner of roast goose, fresh greens, and berries from our Tanunak harvest. The delicious meal soon soothed frayed tempers. At that point it didn't take much to make us happy.

After dinner Dr. Swanson, Dr. Pope, Mrs. Schaubel, Kitty, and I started for shore in the dory. On the way we lost the channel and became mired in the mud flats. Since the tide wouldn't be high enough to float the boat for an hour, and our destination was visible, Kitty and Mrs. Schaubel opted to wade a mile

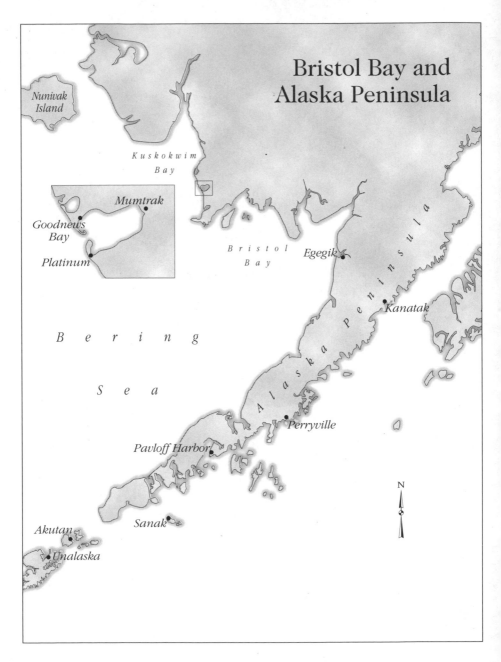

Bristol Bay and
Alaska Peninsula

Bristol Bay had some of the greatest contrasts we encountered. Modern fish canneries and many people who spoke English living practically next door to very primitive villages where most spoke and understood only their own Native language.

through the muck rather than wait for the tide. Platinum, a predominantly white community, had two sections. The small settlement on the coast gave access to a larger town of 80 people at the mine 12 miles back in the hills. The mine had furnished about 90 percent of the platinum that the U.S. had used during the war, and was amazingly sophisticated. Mumtrack, a village only 11 miles up the bay, was amazingly undeveloped. Here we saw an astounding contrast—a traditional Eskimo culture existing only two hours distance from a modern, wealthy community using the latest technical equipment for dredging platinum from the earth.

Kitty's first stop was the post office, where the postmistress, Mrs. Harwood, handed her a large bundle of accumulated mail awaiting our arrival. At last we would have news of our families.

When the doctors and I reached shore, Mr. Neil Hansen, the storekeeper, was waiting to drive us into town. We dried off and warmed up with hot coffee in his cozy and beautifully furnished home. We met most of the white residents—they just happened to drop in. The clean, neat, and well-stocked store, the beautiful houses, and a greenhouse all resembled a small town in the States. Dr. Swanson made the usual arrangements for our program with the various villages of the area.

Monday it blew again, and it was unlikely that anyone would be coming for X-rays. Kitty went down in the fo'c'sle to give Johnny some medicine. The boat gave a lurch, she slipped, fell the length of the ladder, and landed flat on the floor. She felt shaken, but it was not until she climbed back up and turned to step on the deck that she realized she had injured her knee. Dr. Swanson said she had pulled the ligaments, and that with the constant rolling of the ship, the only way to secure it was with a plaster cast, which he and Mrs. Schaubel applied.

At first Kitty did not like the idea of a cast, but soon she was grateful for the support and security it gave her. Fortunately, no patients came during the time that Kitty had to be quiet while the cast dried. She had a few hours of complete rest. Then it was back to work on board the ship, while Mrs. Schaubel did the village work with the doctor.

Kitty and I laughed when we remembered our worries about what kind of a doctor would replace Dr. Schwinge. We thanked God for Dr. Swanson. He had an easy-going personality and was conscientious and knowledgeable about his work. His experience on fishing boats in Southeast Alaska meant that he knew his way around on the water. But he was worrying about being so out of touch with his wife during the last part of her pregnancy and was eager to finish the trip and return to her.

A nearby airfield made it possible to transport Johnny to Bethel, where Dr. Swanson made arrangements for him to be properly cared for in the hospital. With Kitty in a cast and a busy week ahead, no one would be able to give him the care he needed down in the fo'c'sle. In addition, Dr. Swanson could not predict how long Johnny would be ill. Even the most prejudiced crew members felt sorry for him by the time he left, looking pale and frightened. They realized that he had stoically suffered a great deal of pain from the disease, exacerbated by the constant rolling of the ship. We would miss this intelligent and hard-working young man with his friendly, cheerful disposition and good-natured explanations of Eskimo customs.

Johnny's illness and Kitty's fall made us think—we were out in the middle of nowhere, often with no communication with the outside world for days at a time. In the event of any serious health problem, transportation to a hospital would be difficult—and in addition we wondered if any emergency messages from home would ever catch up with us. This worry was heavy on Dr. Swanson's mind and on mine.

Dr. Swanson and Mrs. Schaubel made the two-hour trip in the dory to the Eskimo town of Mumtrack, where they met Mr. and Mrs. Hoffman, the schoolteachers. The condition of these local youngsters was deplorable. Almost every one had scabies, and the majority had secondary infections. The children spoke very little English and were unable to understand what we told them, though adults spoke some English. The village had been without a school since 1937, until this year.

These Eskimos had little contact with Platinum. They were reluctant to travel the 10 miles of protected water by outboard to the *Hygiene*. On one home visit, Dr. Swanson found a four-year-old boy ill with pneumonia. The child had been sick for 10 days, and the parents had made no effort to contact Dr. Wareham at Platinum, who later told Dr. Swanson he would like to help cases such as this. The people of Mumtrack were apathetic and as out of touch as those of Mekoryuk, and lacked in addition the benefit of a reindeer plant to help their economy.

After four days, we essentially completed our work, but we could not leave because our fuel tanks were almost empty. An oil freighter was due any day, so we waited three days for it. During the delay, Dr. Wareham invited us for lunch in the mining camp mess-hall and gave us a tour of the camp and the dredging operation. He showed us the draglines and hydraulic giants. Powerful jets of water washed the gravel into sluice boxes, where the riffles caught the platinum. Everywhere huge bulldozers were shoving piles of gravel around. An immense 90-bucket dredge sat in its own lake. I could not imagine how they had transported all this massive equipment to this remote location.

The doctor ended our tour in the company office, where many large platinum nuggets were on display. He let me hold a quart jar containing the previous day's cleanup of $30,000. With the help of willing arms and crutches, Kitty was able to make most of the trip, and found that her cast did not hinder her too much.

Many of the people working at the mine had an interest in the place—they either owned some of the claims or were relatives of the owners. As we walked along, the doctor introduced me to a kid in dirty overalls who was carrying a shovel. He was the owner's brother, and both were millionaires.

Then he drove us around to show off the model camp. About a fourth of the miners lived there with their families in well-kept, comfortable homes. Lettuce, celery, cabbage, and radishes, all of amazing size, filled the neat vegetable gardens and made our mouths water. The rest of the workers lived in comfortable barracks.

By contrast, the people in Goodnews and Mumtrack lived on berries and fish. They offered us one of their delicacies, which they prepared by burying a fish vertically, head down, in a hole in the ground with just the tip of its tail visible. When the fish had rotted enough so they could pull the backbone out by the tail, they considered it perfect for eating. This treat did not make our mouths water.

In Platinum I discovered that I had gone to the University of Washington with Hal Hansen, son of the couple who ran the store. From then on, the Hansens' house was open to me whenever I could stop in. I was able to do my laundry and, glory be, I had two showers in one week. The Hansens had a greenhouse filled with fresh vegetables, which they offered me— what bliss! When the ship had been at St. Lawrence Island, I had commented several times that I would not mind being left there, but I had to admit the niceties of civilization looked awfully good to me in Platinum.

As we continued to wait for fuel, we took advantage of the sunny weather to go ashore, where we picked berries and enjoyed moving around on solid ground. The movie "State Fair," showing at the Skookum Kashim, the mining camp theater, provided a pleasant diversion from our health films. The next evening we bowled at the recreation center. It seemed like Saturday night in the big city. The enforced delay at Platinum gave us all a much-needed respite, and tensions subsided.

During this interlude Dr. Pope cut his first head of hair, and Dr. Swanson was his first victim. After a month's growth, Dr. Swanson had claimed he could not hear well, and finally decided to risk the operation. We thought the results indicated that Dr. Pope might be a better barber than dentist.

Because of the extremely high incidence of scabies with secondary infections, Mrs. Schaubel planned to stay and continue caring for the people in the two villages for a week or so after the *Hygiene* left. She also hoped to get in touch with some of the villagers with TB who had left Mumtrack and Goodnews, contrary to instructions, for their fishing camps. We would have liked to shanghai this good-looking, gray-haired vigorous nurse, but Dr. Swanson was sure the ANS would disapprove. Her dedication to her people in the remote villages in this vast area was awe-inspiring.

We were eager to get on with the work as soon as we could get fuel. The storms were coming more and more frequently, and the *Hygiene* was supposed to be out of the Bering Sea by September 1, only a week away. Finally the oil barge came alongside, and we took on fuel and a few drums of water, then left Goodnews Bay for Egegik. We deleted Togiak from our schedule because we had been told that the villagers were at widely scattered fishing camps this time of year.

Egegik
Tuesday, August 26, to Friday, August 29

Two hours out of Platinum the port engine stopped. We still made headway, but slowly. Gus discovered that one of the high-pressure fuel lines had broken. He, Wendell, and Dr. Pope made temporary repairs, and after a few hours were able to get the engine going again. Fortunately the sea was relatively calm and the visibility fair.

Captain Kippola had been unable to find a replacement for Johnny at Platinum, so the next morning I was on the bridge again. A drifting fog gave us occasional glimpses of the mountains of the Alaska Peninsula. I was surprised how reassuring it was to see a definite land mass instead of the broad plain of half-land, half-water. Captain Kippola placed the ship about 10 miles from Egegik. He proceeded slowly, because of the shallow and muddy water. At 10:30 a.m. he dropped the anchor about six miles out, after briefly seeing a light where Egegik should have been. Then the fog again blotted out the shoreline.

After lunch, John, Dr. Swanson, Kitty, and I, with our shore kits, started out in the dory aiming for the occasionally visible light on the northern shore of the bay. John had a chart, but it was no help—the channels all looked alike. We meandered around the sandspits trying to find and follow the main watercourse of the large Egegik River. Again and again John headed up a promising channel that dead-ended, sometimes suddenly, sometimes after a mile or two. Buildings were visible on the shore whenever the fog lifted, but the *Hygiene* had disappeared. Trapped in a maze, we speculated on what it would be like to spend the night in an open boat on the cold, damp sea. At last John hit the right slot, and we reached the town after four hours of wandering around, grateful that the wind had not come up while we searched for the correct passage.

Dr. Swanson contacted the teacher, Mrs. Peter Dakulak, and the cannery superintendent to plan our program and transportation. Mr. Davis, the cannery boat manager, thought it would be best if he sent a pilot out to bring the ship to within a mile of the cannery. He even offered to fly Dr. Swanson out if the fog lifted. Dr. Swanson left John and Mr. Davis to work out the details and went back to a clinic for the school children. We were back in Aleut country, and the children in the village appeared more white than Aleut, displaying a variety of racial traits including African-American, Aleut, and white.

While we worked, the fog became more dense, making it impossible for the pilot or anyone else to go out to the *Hygiene* that evening. Again we were marooned ashore. This time the cannery crew fed us a fine meal in the mess hall. They gave Kitty and me bunks in an empty dormitory, while John and the doctor spent the night aboard the power barge to be on hand at 6 a.m., when the pilot planned to leave for the *Hygiene*.

The town had two canneries. Both were shutting down for the winter. Quite a few white "outsiders" had spent the summer there, and they welcomed our new faces. Consequently Kitty and I had many invitations to the movie, "mug-ups," and ice cream from an ice-cream machine, a real treat after months with none.

The next morning Mr. Davis and his assistant, nicknamed "Sad Sack," aroused the doctor and John, and they left in the fog for the *Hygiene*, running aground twice with the shallow-draft *Snow Bird*. Breakfast was being served when they arrived. The pilot advised Captain Kippola to start for Egegik immediately, to take advantage of the rising tide. Even with a 15-foot tide, the *Hygiene's* keel scraped bottom outside Coffee Point before they dropped anchor at six fathoms, a mile from the cannery.

The people of Egegik were eager for dental and medical services. By late afternoon we had X-rayed and examined the majority of the townspeople. Most were from Egegik, although two families were from Kanatak, a small village on the Kodiak Island side of the Alaska Peninsula, and a few men were from Pilot Point and Naknek.

English was the predominant language here, which made our work much easier. The doctor and Kitty were happy to find a town where the residents could read the pre-natal and infant care brochures they distributed. People lived in clean, comfortably furnished, well-built frame houses that had several rooms. Despite the higher standard of living, we found that 20 of the 96 people we X-rayed had suspicious survey films. Again venereal disease was prevalent; we had not seen any cases during the past month.

At 10 p.m. Captain Kippola moved the ship to the sturdy Alaska Packers dock, tying her securely because she would be aground when the tide was out. We took on water and fuel and stayed there for the next few days. We thus could do laundry, shower, and freely come and go from the ship, but we had no electricity whenever the tide was out. Therefore we had to squeeze X-raying, clinic hours, and meals into the periods of high tide.

Dr. Swanson and Kitty moved their record work onto the deck. I set my microscope on a small table and tried to examine the slides using sunlight. That was not efficient because the sun kept moving. The ship was festooned with laundry flying in the breeze. Unfortunately, the unpleasant smell of a cannery beach after a busy season surrounded us.

We finished our work in the early evening. Dr. Swanson hoped to leave on the night high tide, but a strong southwest wind blew in and kept us at the dock. We prayed for the wind to die during the evening, because if we could not get out on the next high tide, we might be delayed in Egegik for a week.

Captain Kippola asked a family who had come from Pilot Point by small boat how many people were there. They said the people had scattered widely after the cannery closed and few people would be there, so Dr. Swanson decided to delete Pilot Point from the schedule. We would leave the Bering Sea with no time to spare, as the date was now August 30.

It was here that Dr. Pope began charging for his dental services and his decision was questioned. But Dr. Pope assured everyone that he should and would charge fees, and the money would be returned to the Health Department.

Akutan
Sunday, August 31, to Monday, September 1

We headed for Akutan through rough seas. The boat pranced and jumped in the choppy water, making it impossible for Jessie to cook or for anyone to work. Even a moderate wind in the shallow waters of the area caused rough seas. I kept busy standing wheel watches with the captain. I enjoyed helping on the bridge, but I soon realized that working the extra 12 hours a day was making me very tired, especially when the weather was bad.

At noon on Sunday we approached Akutan Island. Tide rips around some of the points gave us an even greater bouncing than we had been experiencing. At 2:30 p.m. the weary crew dropped anchor in one of the most picturesque, well-defined harbors we had yet visited. The definite beach, only 100 yards away, seemed like paradise after anchorages four and five miles out from an indistinct and sometimes invisible shore.

The pleasure of reaching paradise soon evaporated when Dr. Swanson and Dr. Pope asked Gus to start the generator so we could begin working immediately. For the first time since I had been on the ship, I rebelled. Kitty and Gus joined in, maybe even angrier than I was. We all refused to work that afternoon. An excerpt from one of my letters described our feelings;

> As soon as we dropped the anchor in this beautiful little bay and stopped rolling for the first time in two days Dr. Swanson and Dr. Pope asked Gus to start the generator for the X-ray machine. They wanted to get things going even before we ate. Gus was tired because he had been working the last two days and so had I. We felt that since this was Sunday and we were supposed to have Sundays off, it wouldn't hurt, under the circumstances, to have at least a part of the afternoon off. Tomorrow is Labor Day and we will be happy to work then but right now we are *tired* and *hungry*.
>
> We have made it out of the Bering Sea on schedule. We have worked as hard and as long as necessary all summer and have not considered hours at all, often working till two or three in the morning, if it was necessary. We have done it willingly and cheerfully as the need was obvious. The Popes are very angry at our refusal to work this Sunday afternoon. They are bored and want to go home. We feel we are justified in our actions and they can go to blazes. There, I got that off my chest.

While the crew, Kitty, and I ate, rested, and wrote letters, Dr. Swanson and Dr. Pope went ashore in a dory that came out to meet the ship. They met the teachers, Mr. and Mrs. Archie Paine, at the schoolhouse, where they set up a clinic and made up the X-ray cards for the 58 residents.

We heard later that they gorged themselves at Mrs. Paine's fine supper table. Dr. Swanson remarked it must have looked as though they had not eaten in days. None of us had eaten a hot substantial meal since we left Egegik, because the roll of the ship made cooking and serving meals almost impossible.

Our work went smoothly and quickly on Monday morning. Everyone spoke and understood English. Akutan's population was one of the several villages that had been evacuated to Southeast Alaska during the threatened Japanese invasion of the Aleutians. We had essentially completed our program by 4 p.m. Dr. Swanson would hold conferences in the morning. This was the first village in the area with a low incidence of TB.

When dinner was over, I climbed down the ladder and dropped into my kayak to join Kitty, Gus, and some of the other crew members, who were in the rowboat. They wanted to explore the bay, especially the remains of an old whaling station. As I paddled in my stable, comfortable kayak, slightly separated from the others, I imagined how happy the old whalers must have felt coming into this snug harbor with its calm waters. The setting sun brilliantly highlighted the white buildings. Soon the full moon came up. It was a night for romance. Kitty and Gus again looked as though they might be thinking of more than just being shipmates. We had been so busy and tired the last few months that they had hardly seen each other. Now they seemed to have a great deal to discuss.

The McGlashen family invited us ashore, where we enjoyed coffee and cake that they just happened to be serving. The fine, clean homes of the community impressed us as we walked through the village on our way to the schoolhouse to show the slides for "It Can Be Done," on home care for tuberculosis.

Following the showing, we joined the townspeople at a dance unlike any other we had attended. At first most of the people were at the schoolhouse, and the music went along at a normal pace. As more and more people went home and turned on their lights, the music became slower and extremely sedate. But midnight approached, and the more sensible members of the community turned out their lights and went to sleep. Each time a light went out more electrical power was delivered to the record player in the schoolhouse—the music increased in speed until we looked like whirling dervishes and collapsed in heaps of breathless laughter.

At noon we weighed anchor for Unalaska, and at 5 p.m. we tied up at a dock. Except for Egegik, it was the first time we had been able to get on and off the ship conveniently since entering the Bering Sea, and this gave us a delicious sense of freedom. What had seemed the end of the world on the *Hygiene's* way north was now civilization.

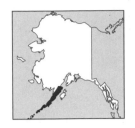

Alaska Peninsula

Unalaska
Tuesday, September 2, to Saturday, September 6

It did not take long to learn the disadvantages of docking near the Dutch Harbor Navy base. That evening, as the last liberty boat was ready to return to the Navy base across the channel, rowdy young sailors set up a wild clamor around the float where we were moored. They had many teenage Aleut girls in tow. The girls soon dispersed back to their homes on the departure of the liberty launch. The residents of the village were understandably reluctant to venture out after dark because of the invasion of the inevitable drunks. Unalaska appeared to be a village disorganized by more than its share of carousing sailors.

Mr. Robinson, the city marshal, helped get word around that we were ready to work. The turnout was poor, and the enthusiasm we had seen in June on our way north had disappeared. The town had lost its public health nurse in the spring. She left following a controversy over an investigation of venereal disease. It was certain that the town needed the full-time services of a public health nurse.

After November 1947 the Navy planned to withdraw its medical personnel, and Unalaska would have no medical services. Considering that the town had a hospital and served an isolated scattered population located in a remote area, it was logical a medical center should remain there. Dr. Swanson advised the village leaders to make a direct written appeal to the Alaska Department of Health for a nurse. He told them that they should know the specific duties of a public health nurse. If, in line of duty, the nurse recommended an action contrary to an individual patient's wishes, that the town would support that recommendation—for example, control of a syphilitic prostitute. It would be essential for the town to back the nurse's recommendations.

At the moment Unalaska boasted three physicians and two dentists. They were all serving on ships temporarily in port. We X-rayed the crews from the *North Star* and the *Aleutian Mail*. The latter was the much-needed mail boat that had just been put into service and ran from Seward along the Peninsula to Unalaska, west to Atka, and then back again.

Four bars and three liquor stores now choked Unalaska, once a thriving Aleut village. Many of the residents commented on the loss of their community spirit. Surrounded as they were by the Navy base exuding the white culture's prosperity and waste, they had difficulty retaining their own more conservative culture. The village leaders hoped that when the base closed in the fall and the liquor stores moved, Unalaska might regain some of its old spirit.

One evening we were invited for dinner at the Civilian Club in Dutch Harbor, where we met some of the people responsible for the final closing of the base. Later a couple of the officers of the *North Star,* which carried a doctor and sometimes a public health nurse, invited us to go on an inspection tour of their ship. The Natives had often referred to the help given them by the *North Star,* so we felt it was an old friend and were happy to be able to visit.

While we were having coffee in the officers' mess, we heard a commotion outside the door. Suddenly it burst open, and one of the crewmen came in swinging a knife and cursing: enraged because the officers could invite women to the ship when he could not. Several other men were trying to stop him as he moved, knife flashing, to attack the officers. He was very strong, and out of his mind. Finally the men wrestled the knife away from him before he hurt anyone. He refused to calm down, so they put him in the town jail. The situation was frightening and quite embarrassing. Kitty and I were upset that we had been the cause of such a scene.

We lost another valuable crew member at Dutch Harbor, and again the captain could find no one to replace him. Old John Bergquist, our mate, left the ship. We knew we would miss him, not only when it came to ship operations, but for his fine spirit and companionship.

We moved around to the Dutch Harbor oil dock on Saturday morning to take on fuel and water. This was a big day for Kitty. Dr. Swanson took the cast off her knee. She had become very adept at swinging the awkward thing around, but it definitely put a cramp in her style. She said she missed its support, but in a couple of hours her knee again felt normal. To celebrate, she and Gus took the ferry back to Unalaska to pick up laundry they had left there.

That afternoon the wind rose to gale proportions, it blew so much water into the air that the harbor looked smoky, and by 5 p.m. the captain estimated the wind velocity at 40 to 60 mph. Coming back on the ferry, Kitty and Gus compared the howling gale to the William Tell Overture. The men had to put out extra lines to secure the *Hygiene.* Tied to the neighboring dock, the 3000-ton *Unalga* snapped her moorings, and her crew had to put out 15 lines to secure her.

The storm was a small example of what an Aleutian wind could do. It came in gusts, picking up the waves in sheets and flinging them in the air between the two docks, first from one direction and then the other. It tore at our clothes and packages. These phenomena had the local name "williwaw." We could see the many small whirlwinds that sucked water into their centers roaring down the bay. I had difficulty walking against the wind as I went down the dock. One gust was so strong that I sat down and waited for it to go by. I was glad it was not a steady wind of that strength. By early morning the storm abated and we left at 4 a.m. for Sanak.

Sanak and Pavlov Harbor
Sunday, September 7, to Monday, September 8

We made good time with the breeze on our stern and clearing weather. At Scotch Cap we could see the wreck of the SS *Mt. McKinley* on the distant shore. In the early afternoon, visibility was good enough to discern Mt. Shishaldin's smoking peak about 20 miles away.

Sanak's almost landlocked harbor afforded an excellent anchorage. When no one came out from shore, Dr. Swanson asked the captain to lower the dory so he could go in and set up plans for the next day. Up to this point, the captain had wholeheartedly accommodated the demands of the program. This time he rebelled. He said that he and his men had been working since 4 a.m. and that was long enough. He would be happy to take the doctor ashore in the morning.

After the captain and crew went into the dining salon for their turn at dinner, Dr. Swanson grumbled that this would cause at least a half-day's delay. I volunteered, "If you can put my kayak in the water, I'd be happy to paddle in, get the census, and deliver the needed information." I thought that would be a good excuse to go for a paddle. The doctor and dentist quickly lowered the ship's ladder and set the kayak in the water. With very little surf breaking, I thought it would be a great adventure.

Darkness was approaching rapidly by the time I had settled in my cockpit. I began to feel it might not be such a simple paddle after all, particularly when I moved a short distance from the ship and heard a wave crash close to me. The crew and captain were eating and unaware of what was going on.

The beach was about a third of a mile away. Periodically waves broke over submerged rocks. It grew dark rapidly. I couldn't see the rocks till white foam boiled up, although I could hear the breaking waves, and occasionally I would be frightened by one erupting unexpectedly next to me.

I began to realize that I was being foolhardy. Captain Kippola had sound reasons for not sending a small boat to shore through unknown waters in the dark. I decided to keep going, since someone had built a fire on the beach around which people were milling. I called for help to land and several flashlights pointed to the safest area. By that time, rocks were scattered everywhere, and I was afraid of puncturing my kayak. Voices directed me to the proper channel, and when I reached shore many willing hands pulled me up the beach.

Two schoolteachers, an older woman and a handsome young man, greeted me. They had arrived the day before and were enjoying a beach fire and meeting the people of their communities. "We haven't had a chance to read our mail and didn't know who you were," they explained.

The woman looked at me and shook her head, "I don't believe it. A blond young lady. And you paddled a kayak here in the dark? I was sure you were an Eskimo fisherman." We sat around the fire a few minutes while I answered their questions. "Where did you get the kayak? Were you afraid paddling in the dark?" I had to admit I was, and then explained my mission. Dick, the younger teacher from Pavlov, arranged for one of the Aleuts to take Mrs. West, the teacher from Sanak, himself, and me back to the *Hygiene* in his boat, which had an outboard and a searchlight. They towed the little kayak safely behind.

On our return, Captain Kippola, looking very stern, took me aside and gravely admonished, "Susie, I've trusted you with your kayak and you've been cautious. But this episode was just plain stupid. From now on you are not to take your kayak off the ship without my permission. Is that understood?"

I felt like a teenager being grounded, but I had to admit I deserved it. I replied, "Yes—I realized when I was halfway in that I was doing a dumb thing. I got scared, but—well, I thought it would be safer to keep going than to turn back."

"Did the doctor ask you to go?"

"No, it was my idea. I was just trying to be helpful and—well, I always like an excuse to go for a paddle."

Only later did I learn that when the captain came out from dinner and found out what was going on, he was so furious that he started a fistfight with the dentist, and the men had to forcibly separate them. Kitty told me that as I disappeared in the darkness, even the doctor had some qualms about the whole escapade. They were relieved when I returned with the teachers.

Sanak Island had a population of about 40, divided into two communities, Sanak and Pavlov Harbor, They were about 10 miles apart, and each had its own teacher. With the help of Mrs. West, Sanak's teacher, and Dick, Pavlov's teacher, we made up a census and filled out cards for both towns. Dick arranged to go to Pavlov by boat in the early morning to get his people. That evening we outlined our schedule for the next day.

Somehow in the short time we had that evening, Dick and I discovered that we had a great deal in common. He had gone to the University of Washington about the same time I had. He even had some of the same professors. He was working on a Ph.D. in geography and was apparently as entranced with the blond young lady in the kayak as I was with him. It was the first time on the trip I had fallen in love, except with a boat.

We finished our program in one day, finding only two cases of TB in the entire population. Most of the predominantly white islanders lived in large, neat homes. Mrs. West, a motherly person, offered to board one of the boys whose parents both had TB. The island had a post office, but no store, cannery, or any other commercial enterprise. One family had 18 children. Their mother was an influential member of the school board.

At 5:30 p.m. Dr. Swanson notified the captain that we were finished. By 6:30 we were underway. I was disappointed that we were so efficient at this particular stop. I would have liked an opportunity to spend more time with Dick. As it was, we made a hurried exchange of addresses and promised to write when we could.

Perryville
Tuesday, September 9, to Thursday, September 11

A four-hour run put us in King Cove, where we spent the night at the dock. "A needless stop," Dr. Swanson and the Popes complained. Before he lost two crew members, the captain had consented to run the ship at night so the medical staff could work effectively during daylight hours. But he had been unable to replace either Johnny or Old John, the mate. The crew was overworked and dissatisfied, even though Ronald and I stood wheel watches with the captain and Del. If the ship ran at night, the men still had to maintain it during the day: keep the generators running during the X-raying, help with loading and unloading patients, and run the small boat. This meant that they worked day and night. Captain Kippola had to honor the crew members' time off. He could take no chance of losing any more of them.

The Popes particularly resented not running at night. Mrs. Pope whined constantly about every aspect of shipboard life; she wanted to get back to Juneau as soon as possible. They were so angry they would not speak to anyone except the doctor, or even sit down at the table to eat with us, arriving after everyone else was through. This behavior did not endear them to the galley staff, especially when Ronald was helping in the wheelhouse every spare minute he had. Dr. Swanson was also eager to get back (everyone was), but he was philosophical about it and understood the need for one day off a week.

Captain Kippola explained to Dr. Swanson and Dr. Pope that now that the ship was out of dangerous waters, he planned to work reasonable hours. Most ships had three watches, so each person could work eight hours a day. The *Hygiene* had only two watches, which meant that each crew member put in 12 hours a day, when we had a full crew. This accounted for the difficulty of finding crew replacements.

We had planned only two stops along the Alaska Peninsula. One was Perryville, where we had found so many positive cases the previous year, and the other was Kanatak, which we had skipped the year before because of weather. At Perryville, Mr. Petmickey, the ANS teacher, arrived aboard, upset because no one had warned him the *Hygiene* was coming, although his radio was in good working condition, and he was able to contact Sanak, Unalaska, King Cove, and all other stations along the Peninsula. This was a most unfortunate oversight on the part of the doctor and captain. Such lack of communication was inexcusable, and did not encourage cooperation from the teachers or townspeople. The men of the village were scattered at three fish camps, each several hours distant. Messengers were sent to notify them the *Hygiene* was there.

Dr. Swanson and Kitty noticed a strange reserve among the Natives they talked to. Kitty said they were not the happy people who had welcomed us the year before. Little by little, we learned of the town's disappointment. None of the seven active cases we discovered the previous year had been hospitalized, and two had died. One was the wife of Emil, the town leader who had been so helpful in September of 1946. Mr. Petmickey said that after the *Hygiene's* first stop, the villagers had besieged him for days and months with questions about the forthcoming hospitalization, but it never happened. Just a short time before our present visit, one man had set off with his family in the vain hope of forcing his way into the hospital at Seward.

While Kitty and the doctor showed films, several men, who had been drinking heavily, disturbed the program. Again we heard tales of the mail boat peddling liquor. At the close of the movies, the messengers who had gone to the fish camps returned, bringing very few people back with them.

Three of the active cases we had discovered the year before were at Humpback Bay and refused to leave. Their reasoning was that last year we told them they had TB, and they thought that the government was going to do something for them. The health department had authorized hospitalization and transportation for several patients the previous winter, but the only transportation, the mail boat, had burned and was not replaced for months. The patients felt they were cheated of treatment.

Paradoxically, one far-advanced case of TB actually got into the Seward Sanitarium by a rather roundabout way. The man had been jailed in Kodiak, where the local health nurse, recognizing he had TB and was dangerous to other inmates, had him removed to the sanitarium. This patient died there. So in the minds of the villagers, especially those afflicted with TB, the specter of the disease was made even more gruesome by the fact that the only person they knew who had been treated died instead of being cured.

Kitty and I felt utter discouragement about the situation. We knew, even with the expanded program, that it was not possible to take care of the large number of TB cases we on the *Hygiene* had discovered. We knew it had to be a long-range program. This was difficult to explain to someone whose mother, father, or child had just died. It would have made such a difference if one or two people from each village could have been hospitalized and had begun to recover. When Kitty tried to explain the problem, Emil, who had lost his wife, just looked at her as though to say "words, just words." We found this attitude in all villages we had previously visited. People left so they wouldn't be around for another X-ray survey. They were disillusioned and said they felt like the government had forgotten them.

The new mail boat made a major change because it called on these villages every two weeks instead of every three or four months. Mrs. Petmickey explained that was both good and bad. It took away the total isolation, and we hoped the more readily available transportation and hospital beds would dispel some of the cynicism after a few people were treated and cured. On the other hand, the mail boat made liquor readily available, and with it came a whole new set of problems.

One day the Petmickeys invited Dr. Swanson, Kitty, and me for lunch and served us bear meat that was far more delicious than some we had previously eaten. Mr. Petmickey explained that it was necessary to remove all the fat for the meat to taste sweet. Mrs. Petmickey encouraged us to try some cranberries put up the Aleut way for winter storage. We were a bit hesitant when she described the process. She had placed the berries in a barrel with water, and allowed a mold to form on top as protection for those at the bottom. To our surprise, the slightly moldy taste was delicious.

Kanatak
Friday, September 12, to Saturday, September 13

We reached Kanatak in fine weather and anchored within 200 yards of shore. The community nestled in a green valley between towering mountains, and a bright stream tumbled into the ocean beside it. The boarded-up school and typically unpainted houses made it look deserted, but in fact four small families totaling 20 people lived there. Two families were putting up salmon at Lake Becharof for the winter, and one of the men agreed to hike over to the lake to get them.

Dr. Swanson and Kitty recognized one family that they had seen when we were at Egegik, a nine-mile walk across the peninsula from Kanatak. In Egegik the family had shared a crowded, cluttered shack with others. Their daughter, who had an active case of TB, was jammed in with the rest of the children. Kitty and the doctor were pleasantly surprised to find that in Kanatak, the family's house was clean, and the children were bathed and well behaved. The husband had built a partition around his daughter's bed to isolate her from the rest of the family. It was a bright spot for Kitty, in view of the disillusionment we found in Perryville. She saw that sometimes advice given in the most hopeless situations could bear fruit.

An interesting character at Kanatak was John, a tall, husky white man, who expressed his concern to Kitty about Sophie, a 10-year-old girl whose stepfather was mistreating her. John thought she should be put in a foster home. Kitty said she would refer the problem to the public health nurse in Kodiak.

John told us that 10 years earlier the Standard Oil Company had come in and drilled and capped a number of oil wells. He still had faith and stakes in the wells. But now, overgrown roads and buildings in all stages of collapse made us feel we were in a ghost town.

With ideal conditions, we finished our work by noon. Dr. Swanson suggested taking the rest of the afternoon off while we awaited the return of the messenger. Dr. Swanson, Kitty, and Peggy, plus some of the crew members hiked up the trail leading to the summit of the mountain, an old volcano. They described how its crater now mirrored a blue lake. In the distance they could see Lake Becharof, which the Natives crossed to reach the Bristol Bay canneries. Looking down from the pass onto Lake Becharof, they could not see anyone approaching so they concluded that the families were not coming.

While the rest were hiking, I obtained permission from the captain to take my kayak in to explore the stream flowing out of a nearby lake. The little river was quite swift, and three of the young Aleut boys who had been admiring my

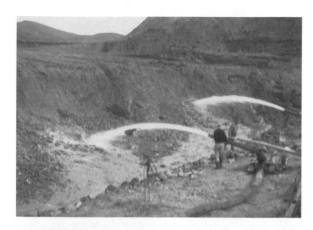

Top: Platinum.
Middle: left, Susie with her
fish, caught in Kanatak;
right, tide out at Egegik.
Bottom: Kanatak Eskimo
boys admire Susie's
kayak.

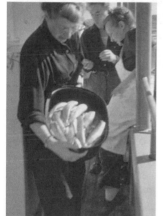

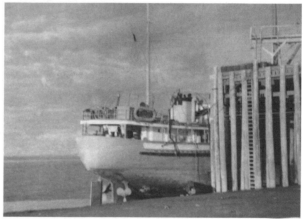

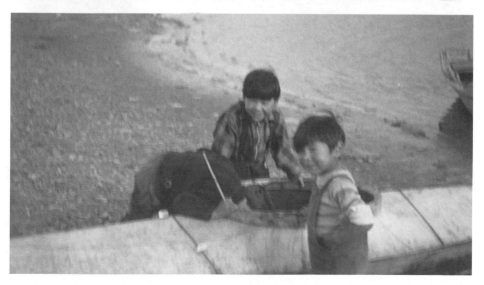

kayak took the bow-line and pulled me up some of the faster sections; otherwise I would never have made it against the current. Coming down was fun and exciting. The current grabbed the kayak, and when I looked down through the clear water I could see the rocks zipping by beneath me at an exciting speed, with no effort on my part except to steer. Swooshing out into the ocean through the breakers, I felt perfectly secure in the little skin boat.

Many salmon fighting upstream to spawn directed my attention to trout feeding on the brilliant orange salmon eggs clustered along the banks. I paddled back to the *Hygiene* for my fishing line and returned to the beach. I figured I might get wet, but it was a warm, sunny day and I wanted to try a sideways landing in the surf the way the big umiaks did on St. Lawrence Island. I waited for one of the larger waves and rode in on a crest about three feet high. The water was breaking and boiling all around the boat as it swung me sideways. I could feel it on my seat through the skin of the kayak. The wave carried me far up the beach, where I hopped out and dragged my trusty little boat high and dry before the next big wave arrived. I knew the captain and some of the other crew members, who had no faith in the kayak, were watching from the ship, sure I would tip over.

The boys who had pulled me up the river earlier met me at the beach full of questions. The oldest asked, "Can I get in your kayak?" I said, "Sure" and handed him the paddle. He sat there having a grand time while pretending he was paddling.

"Do you go out in your father's kayak?" I asked.

"No, he don't have one like this, no one does here, but he tells us stories about them in the old days."

When the children were through playing in the kayak they showed me the trail to a little bridge that crossed the river, where I started to fish. This was the kind of fishing I had expected ever since I had come to Alaska. Every time I put an egg on my hook and dropped it in the water another big Dolly Varden hit it. In less than an hour I had stacked 12 of the beauties beside me. A little Native boy who had been fishing with me gave me the 10 he had caught, and we staggered back to the beach with 22 big trout.

The rest of our group had built a bonfire on the shore and had brought supplies for a picnic. When Dr. Swanson and Ronald saw my fish, they borrowed my gear and rushed over to the river to try their luck. In a few minutes they returned with six more beauties. This bounty far exceeded anything we had seen in other fishing holes. Around the campfire, after a half-day of pleasurable activities, we were in high spirits. As darkness fell, Kitty and Gus were suspiciously close to one another. Again I felt something interesting was going on. I wished, as we watched a spectacular display of Northern Lights, that I could have had a night like that on Sanak Island with my new friend, Dick.

On Sunday Dr. Swanson delayed our departure until mid-morning in case the people at the fish camp changed their minds and returned for X-rays. We enjoyed a leisurely breakfast of fried trout, while tantalizing odors of baking blueberry pies drifted out of the galley. Jessie and some of the men had spent the previous afternoon picking the wild blueberries. Our craving for fresh food had almost become an obsession.

In this peaceful atmosphere, Dr. Swanson, Captain Kippola, Kitty, and I sat around the table discussing the best course to follow for the rest of the trip. Captain Kippola suggested we should go directly to Cook Inlet while the weather was relatively good. Then we could backtrack to Kodiak Island, which we could circle almost any time of the year.

While sympathetic to the captain's suggestions, Dr. Swanson felt locked into going around Kodiak Island as scheduled. He had sent letters to the villages, and notified the Alaska Native Service nurse of our approximate arrival date in Karluk, where she was to meet us.

Again we were running about a month late. If we had known about the weather, anchorages, and population shifts of the Eskimos living around the Bering Sea, if we had known that we could go through Unimak Pass in May, and if we had known we could work in the Bristol Bay area in early June while the weather was good and the people were in their villages, we could have gained a month of good weather. Then we could have moved north to Norton Sound and St. Lawrence Island after the ice broke. But it was necessary to live through a trial trip in order to make better plans for the future.

Local plans for development and the resulting population increases along the Alaska Peninsula made it imperative to establish health service centers in the area, possibly using Unalaska and the Sand Point cannery hospital. Dr. Swanson hoped the future budget would allow for these new medical facilities. Much of the disillusioned attitude we found in Perryville and along the Alaska Peninsula might have been prevented had there been a readily available itinerant nurse.

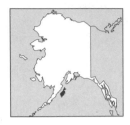

Kodiak Island

Karluk, Larsen's Bay, and Alitak
Monday, September 15, to Saturday, September 20

We continued the plan to circle Kodiak Island, stopping at the towns we had serviced the previous year and picking up villages we had missed. The trip would be much shorter than that of the year before, because we had identified most of the cases and done the preliminary work. Margaret Gunn, the new ANS nurse for Kodiak Island, joined us at Karluk. She was a bright and enthusiastic young lady from New England, full of fun, who reminded us of Katharine Hepburn.

The trip around Kodiak Island was not happy. The captain and the doctors were again in constant conflict. Both Dr. Swanson and Dr. Pope worried we would not be able to get out of Cook Inlet if we didn't move faster. Captain Kippola was sticking to his plan of not traveling at night and taking Sundays off. He was doing his best to keep the crew happy, and did not want to lose anyone in Kodiak; he still had two crew positions to fill.

As the time of our arrival in Kodiak drew near, the crew dreamed of the bars and stores. They also became more and more concerned and angry because no one had received a paycheck for two months. Rumors spread around the ship—that the Health Department had run out of money, or they weren't going to pay anyone till we returned to Juneau, and so on. Those who lived from paycheck to paycheck and were out of money were unhappy at the thought of being broke in Kodiak.

Conditions were no better on shore. We continued to feel a distinct coldness and cynicism in all the villages we had visited earlier. People did not show up for X-rays or clinics. Again and again we heard them comment, "What's the use?" We noticed much more drunkenness and continued to hear claims that the liquor came on the mail boat. One patient complained that Dr. Pope had refused to give her dental care because she could not pay for it.

One morning while we were working at Alitak, a plane landed on the beach. The pilot brought a large bag of mail, including paychecks. He explained that Miss Curtis, the nurse in Kodiak, thought it might boost our morale so she asked him to drop it off on one of his trips. She and that pilot were the two best people on Kodiak Island as far as the crew of the *Hygiene* was concerned.

After reading letters from his very pregnant wife, Dr. Swanson was more anxious than ever to return to Juneau. Eight letters from my mother, assuring me that all was well, relieved my mind. Even the dental instruments Dr.

Pope had been expecting daily for nearly three months arrived. Parts for the broken engine also arrived, but they were not what Gus had ordered so he couldn't use them.

Alitak had an alarming increase in venereal diseases, particularly syphilis. We found seven new cases since the previous year. At the rate syphilis was spreading just in that one town, the entire adult population and some of the children would be infected by 1951 unless the Territorial Health Department made them eligible for treatment.

Old Harbor
Sunday, September 21, to Friday, September 26

A group of exceptionally jovial young men greeted us on the beach at Old Harbor. We soon realized that they were drunk. The mail boat *Shuyak* had pulled in and disposed of its liquid freight the previous day. We started our usual clinics with the children at the schoolhouse. Kitty noticed that this year, instead of the parents bringing the children to us, elder siblings or grandparents were escorting them.

Following the clinic, Dr. Swanson, Philip Kaguyak, a village leader, and I called at the homes of about 20 people whose X-rays had been positive the year before, and whom we wished to X-ray that afternoon. The villagers' homes were neat and clean, as they had been on our previous visit, but they were quite a contrast to the condition of the occupants many of whom were sleeping off a drunk. The truth soon came out—the village was almost completely downed by liquor. Various people told us conflicting stories of its arrival. Some said the mail boat brought it; others claimed it was flown in. From the looks of the townspeople, it could have been both.

Men and women had passed out on their steps or porches, some along the paths. Babies still nursing were crying from hunger because their mothers were not conscious enough to nurse them. Young teenage girls were trying to care for many of the frightened and hungry little ones.

As they became sober, the people were still reluctant to go to the *Hygiene* for X-rays. In some instances they consented to having their children X-rayed, but it was the same old story—"What is the use?" The next morning, when Dr. Swanson and Miss Gunn went ashore to make house calls, the adults who were then sober still made no effort to get X-rayed.

Immediately Dr. Swanson called a meeting of the community leaders. He introduced Miss Gunn, who was new to the district. Then she and Dr. Swanson discovered the reason for the people's reluctance to avail themselves of the health program. Here, as in Perryville, they were suspicious of and antagonistic to a program that consisted of finding TB by surveys, but which did not treat or hospitalize the ill. In addition, since we had been there the previous year, many villagers had died during a flu epidemic. The village elders had appealed to the public health nurse in Kodiak for help, but had delayed until the epidemic was so far advanced that people were already dead, or nearly so.

Dr. Swanson forcefully and graphically explained that the villagers themselves could do much about improving their health. Their own immediate efforts in caring for their sick at home while they awaited sanitarium care were important, both for their recovery and to prevent further spread of the disease. His talk was simple and to the point, and it brought results. Nearly all of the town turned out for X-rays, and they jammed the schoolhouse to the doors that evening to see the 35mm slide program, "Home Care of TB."

Once the people of the village understood the hazards of a contagious disease spread by germs and the dangers of crowding in their homes, they were cooperative and appreciative. Again we hoped that with follow-up advice and home instruction in caring for the sick, much could be accomplished. Understandably these people's knowledge of infection and the need to isolate illness required constant reinforcement.

In smaller communities, the teachers were a great aid in such a program, particularly in villages where the visits of the nurses were infrequent. Philip told us that when the schoolteachers were there, the liquor supply dried up. The teachers for Old Harbor had not yet arrived for the year but were expected daily.

Eventually we X-rayed all but six residents. One who stayed away was the father of the little boy who had had a far-advanced case of TB the previous year, and who was still very ill. This was the man who had consistently denied that his son was sick. He was also next in line to be village chief. In this capacity he would have a definite influence on his village, and we were concerned because they needed the kind of leadership that would help them control this disease, not ignore it.

After we left Old Harbor, the damaged fuel-injection valve again delayed us. It was leaking badly and running fuel oil into the bilges, so we anchored for the night while the engineers worked on it. The delays were getting on everyone's nerves, and friction seemed the normal state of affairs. Peggy, who had been so obliging at the start, had cabin fever from constantly being on the boat trying to keep up with the typing. She announced, uncharacteristically, "I'm going ashore today to get some pictures in the daylight. I'll type my reports tonight." We wondered who she thought would receive the people, give them their cards, and direct them to the X-ray clinic.

We were not a happy group. Nearly everyone was upset with something or someone on board. In a letter I wrote to my mother I summed up my feelings about the work since we left the Bering Sea.

> The last two weeks have been the most depressing I have experienced on the ship. We have done what we planned, in spite of generator troubles and engine troubles, but when we return to a village, the families of patients who have died or are steadily getting worse ask what good are we doing? Why can't their sick relative be put in a hospital? Even some of the teachers are wondering what we are really doing.
>
> We know that the situation will improve dramatically in a few years, but it is very difficult to explain, that right now we cannot recommend hospitalization for hopeless cases or for those who might be able to recover with home care. Only serious cases with good chances for recovery are even eligible to be considered. The list is so long and the hospital beds so pitifully few that a very small number are chosen, and we don't make the choices.
>
> We have described the new hospital at Sitka and money that has been voted for more beds, but until a member of their community is helped, this is all empty words and promises, and I can't blame them for being bitter and disillusioned. This has been their history. We have to work on the assumption that it will be several years before they have any hope of getting hospital treatment if they are still alive then.
>
> So again, Kitty and Dr. Swanson tell them how to care for themselves at home, how to keep from spreading the disease, what kind of foods to eat and to rest quietly in bed. This all sounds fine and in theory it would work, but they have to support themselves and that is done by going out in the cold and wet, hunting and fishing. They do help one another, but when 20 percent of a town of 100 to 200 is incapacitated this places a heavy burden on those who aren't.
>
> It may be this has hit me hard because I developed a nasty cold that I couldn't shake and I had to keep working while feeling completely rotten. I empathized with those cases of TB and felt how they must suffer while trying to keep going. I am about over the cold now, thank goodness, but I keep imagining how I would feel if I knew it would be like that for years.

The trip to Kodiak was a fast one because Ronald was acutely ill. He had a pain in his side so severe that Dr. Swanson had to give him morphine for relief.

Kodiak
Saturday, September 27, to Tuesday, September 30

After docking, we all dispersed in different directions. Dr. Swanson had Ronald in the hospital by 8:30 a.m. with a tentative diagnosis of a kidney stone. Dr. Johnson, the local physician, corroborated his diagnosis.

Captain Kippola hired two new deckhands: Ed Stice, slender and gregarious, and Fred Mueller, a heavy-set, quietly competent man. Both were in their forties and looked as though they would not be easily upset. The new faces, personalities, and able bodies gave us all a lift.

Luckily for us, a laundry had been added to the town's businesses since our visit the year before. The doctors did not want to stay in Kodiak the three days it would take to have the laundry done, but necessity overrode them. At no time since June 8 had the ship stopped long enough to do more than one set of sheets or towels per person. We had been using the same linens for three weeks at a time. Salt water and mud had impregnated the clothes of those who made shore trips. Kitty tried, but no longer looked the spotless nurse she had been in the past. She commented, "I'm sure going to recommend that we need more linens and planned stops for laundry."

I found a source of fresh milk at 75 cents a quart and bought myself a quart every day, plus fresh melons and ice cream. Jessie refilled her nearly depleted larder. Even the staples and canned goods were mostly gone. Thank goodness the shipping strike was over, and the Kodiak stores were again well supplied.

Gus had given up on ordering a replacement part for the damaged fuel valve. He found a machinist at the Navy base, who made him an exact duplicate of the broken part.

Dr. Swanson met with the medical officers at the Navy base, and they planned a strategy to provide transportation in the future for Miss Gunn, in case she was needed in the outlying villages. They assured Dr. Swanson that she would have transportation when she needed it.

On Sunday Wendell, our assistant engineer, returned from church, elated. "I've found a good home here for the little girl who was being abused in Kanatak," he reported. Dr. Swanson quickly made the official arrangements for the child's foster care. In the past, arguments had arisen that the crew and staff should each tend to their own knitting, but everyone benefited when we all knew something of each other's job.

We worried about leaving Ronald in Kodiak. Just before we left, the good news came that he had passed his kidney stone and would be able to depart with us. We had dreaded the thought of losing his good-natured presence. He was an example to all of us—he never grumbled, did his job with enthusiasm and humor, and then helped the rest of us wherever he could. He had happily stood wheel watches in his spare time. He had filled out X-ray cards and ushered the Natives around. When he returned to the ship, a little pale and subdued, he was surprised at our enthusiastic greeting. He reassured us, "I'm as good as new."

The stop in Kodiak gave us a chance to think and realize again that we were pushing the limits of what could be done, both medically and physically. It had been good to have a break and follow our own interests. We again had a full crew. I was relieved because I was getting very tired, as were the others who were standing extra watches.

While we were at the dock, a Russian ship tied up on the opposite side. A fair percentage of the crew were husky-looking women who smiled and waved from the deck of the ship and made many comments that none of us could understand. They were not allowed off the ship except once, when their officers escorted a large group of them to town to see a movie.

Kitty, who was an enthusiastic photographer, talked Gus, who prided himself on being a frugal Scotsman, into buying a 35mm camera complete with all the gadgets. Kitty kidded, "Dr. Schwinge will be pleased. I guess if I can talk Gus into spending money, anything could happen now." I wasn't exactly sure what that meant.

Miss Gunn left the ship in Kodiak, and again we wished we could kidnap a nurse. In addition to being young, attractive, energetic, and a hard worker, she was easy to get along with. Kodiak Island was lucky to have her. Her report on the mail boat follows.

The *Shuyak* is the mail boat which goes bi-monthly around Kodiak Island. It is the only regular authorized carrier service around the Island. During the winter months, it is the only means of transportation, except by plane.

Accommodations are for six passengers. During the summer months there are four extra bunks on the rear deck. The accommodations for the six passengers are three double-decker bunks with mattresses, never washed, never protected, on which are blankets in apparently the same condition. The sleeping quarters are combined with the galley and its table. There is no partition between. One set of these bunks ranges along the side of the table, off which everyone eats. The lavatory is outside and to one side of the hatchway. No washing facilities were noted.

Traveling on the boat at the time of this visit was a primary Luetic* (syphilitic patient). Her bunk was the lower one beside the table. Her clothing and personal effects were on the table, along with the partially finished break-fast. The fo'c'sle had not been scrubbed or swept for some time, and the air was foul. The skipper did not say how many passengers he had, but that he was full up.

As a regular passenger carrier, it seemed as though the protection and care of the passengers was less than adequate, as well as being a menace to the health of the communities at which this boat stops.

Margaret Gunn PHN,
Ouzinkie, Alaska

*She had been checked in Kodiak previously, and also asked for an examination on the *Hygiene* the morning of the visit.

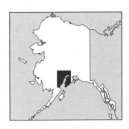

Cook Inlet

Kodiak to Seldovia
Wednesday, October 1, to Friday, October 3

As soon as we left the shelter of Kodiak's harbor, the *Hygiene* began to rock, roll, pitch, and as Kitty said, do everything but turn somersaults. It did not seem possible, but the ship's gyrations increased until we felt as though it was not only standing on end but bending in the middle and snapping back.

Captain Kippola decided the seas were too rough to continue. When he reached the Barren Islands, he found what he thought was a calm anchorage and dropped the hook. The gusts of wind were hitting the boat so hard, however, that the anchor dragged and he decided to move on.

Huge waves hit us beyond the shelter of the islands, The ship rolled so far it felt as if it would turn turtle; the clinometer registered 51 degrees, more than halfway over. The next few minutes were wild. Jessie had started measuring flour, eggs, and some oil for a cake when she thought we were anchoring in a quiet bay. When the ship suddenly moved back into the tumbling water, with no warning, all her supplies out on the counter slid onto the deck and formed a slippery mess. The open flour bin broke loose from its moorings and waltzed around the galley floor in the slimy mixture. Jessie took refuge in a somewhat protected corner and hollered for help.

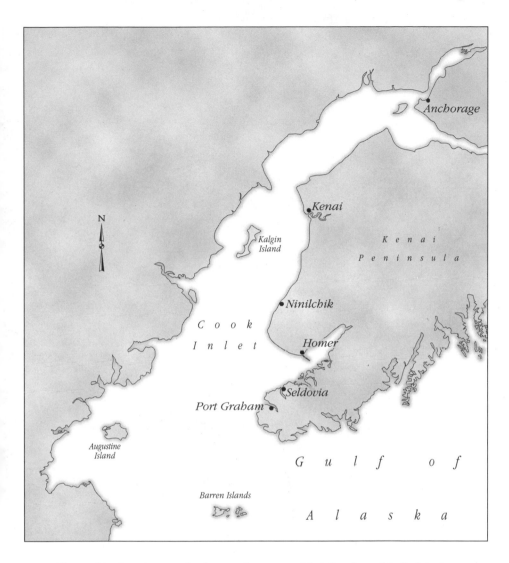

Here white immigrants had started communities they hoped to link to An-chorage by roads. The smaller Native villages were isolated and inhabited by Athapascan Indians, most of whom spoke English. Hospitals were avail-able in the nearby towns of Seldovia, Anchorage and Seward.

Gus came dashing in, took one look at the mess and turned off the oil in the stove. Remembering what had happened the year before, he sent Ronald, who had just appeared, for some two-by-fours to again secure the stove against the wall. All the while the ship was taking tremendous rolls. Jessie went below to regain her composure. Later she reported that some pickled herring Dr. Swanson had collected on the stern took a nose dive down her air vent and landed on her face as she lay in her bunk. Gus told Ronald, "Don't try to clean. Just keep an eye on the stove, I don't think it can go anyplace with that bracing." So the mess continued to mix itself until we crawled into the millpond-calm waters of Port Chatham.

Then began the big clean-up. Not only was the galley a mess, but the clinic had leaked again, and salt water had splattered on everything. I had learned to cover the X-ray equipment with a waterproof tarp, so with luck, it would not have any short circuits. The rest of the clinic was a disaster. Bottles had jumped out of their roll-proof racks, and the deck was covered with broken glass and reagents. The large file cabinet fastened to the wall had pulled loose and tipped over, dumping records into the mess. In addition to these calamities, Gus complained of severe pain in his chest every time he took a breath. Dr. Swanson examined him, said he was suffering from pleurisy, and wound his chest tightly with adhesive tape. This gave Gus some relief. At this point I began to wonder if equipment and personnel were falling apart faster than they could be put back together.

The calm of Port Chatham did not extend into Cook Inlet, so we lay over another day and continued the clean-up. Late in the afternoon, Del and I took the baidarka and kayak and went exploring. The wind and waves caused us a little uneasiness, so we lashed the two boats together, as I had read the Aleuts did in Baranof's time. Then we felt secure. We returned just in time for supper and a surprise birthday cake Jessie had tried to bake for me the day before. I was touched that she went to that effort after all she had been through. Maybe things didn't look so bad after all.

Ninilchik
Saturday, October 4

We picked up Miss Dressler, the new itinerant nurse in Seldovia, and made a fast trip to Ninilchik on the incoming tide. The doctor and nurses set up their clinics at the schoolhouse, which along with the church was high on a hillside above the village. I took X-rays on the ship.

The town was in a good farming area where the settlers were resting their hopes on the new road that was to connect Anchorage and Homer. The site had been settled for many years, and its population combined Polish and Russian whites mixed with Aleuts and Indians. They had intermarried over a long time, and it was impossible to tell anyone's race just by looking. A fairly large group of white bachelors had recently homesteaded.

Mr. Malach, the teacher, said he would be glad when we finished the next day so he could have back his loneliness, lock his doors, and forget all the rush.

The wind came up during the night, and at 6 a.m. the rattle of the anchor chain and the chugging of the engines plus the roll of the ship made us aware that plans had changed. The dory, with the motor still on it, had to be hauled aboard and in the process was almost lost, but was finally safely secured. The captain had heard we were needed at Port Graham, a protected bay, so he headed there.

Port Graham
Sunday, October 5, to Monday, October 6

This village had been added to the itinerary because of the urgent plea of the Cohens, the schoolteachers. The great number of scabies cases, many secondarily infected, justified their request for help. The work was rushed, but later in the month, on an overnight stop, we tied up the loose ends.

I started X-raying, but after a few minutes, the X-ray machine got a case of déjà vu and stopped working for no apparent reason. I told Gus, "I don't think it likes Cook Inlet." Gus and I took everything apart that we could think of, with no results. After four hours of struggle, the machine suddenly worked again, and we had no idea why.

The Cohens entertained us that night with cake and coffee. Mr. Cohen's brother-in-law was the Territorial Treasurer, and he was well acquainted with Territorial programs. They questioned Dr. Pope about his dental fees, asking if this was a new Territorial policy to charge for services, and if indigents had to pay. The latter question had been raised over the care of a patient in whom the Cohens were much interested. Dr. Pope arrogantly explained that he was heading the new Dental Division within the Territory, and that it was going to be his policy that patients pay. He had been charging for his services since we had put in to Egegik. He did say, however, that no patient would be refused care because of indigence.

Kenai and Kasilof
Tuesday, October 7, to Wednesday, October 15

Stopping at Ninilchik on the way to Kenai, we finished the tag-ends of work we had left after our sudden departure three days earlier. People with a variety of ailments needing immediate attention inundated Dr. Swanson. Many patients came for dental work, and Dr. Pope was so busy that for the first time he did not finish until an hour after the medical staff was ready to leave.

We arrived off Kenai just after dark. The ship was to go up the river channel and tie to a dolphin (a cluster of piles) in front of the town. This was tricky, especially because the beacons were not visible. To play it safe, Captain Kippola anchored in the lee of the point.

The next morning we sailed serenely into the river, and the men secured us to the dolphin. The Hudsons, whom we had met at Hoonah earlier, had organized the town and were ready to start when we arrived. Mr. Peterson, the marshal at Unga the previous year, was now at Kenai. It seemed like old-home week. He arranged for two of the local boys to stand by with their dories, so one would always be on shore and one at the ship to transport patients and staff. The waves had thoroughly drenched our dory in the effort to get it aboard during the wind at Ninilchik, and the motor would not run. Other than that, the work was going smoothly, and we were congratulating ourselves on the good weather, organization, and a full crew.

We did not realize, as we were working, that Jessie and Del had been able to get a flight from Kenai into Anchorage, packed their bags, and left without even a goodbye. We felt betrayed and shocked that they would abandon us with no warning or explanation. Fortunately Ed, the deckhand hired in Kodiak, had been cook on the *Kodiak Bear*, and he stepped into the galley with the greatest of ease. His habit of providing a snack at "mug-up" time soon won him an ardent group of enthusiastic supporters. But once again, the captain was short-handed.

Peggy left the next day on a short trip to Anchorage, previously planned and no surprise. Dr. Swanson came down with the pesky cold that had been attacking the ship's personnel one by one. He flew to Kasilof and arranged to have the people of that village flown to Kenai at reduced rates, but only six of the 60 residents took advantage of it. He thought this measure was necessary because of the poor anchorage in front of Kasilof, and because its people were scattered along seven miles of road with no central place of contact.

On Sunday John Monfor, a homesteader, loaded Gus, Kitty, and me in his truck and took us on a sightseeing tour. The scenery was spectacular, the rivers full of fish, the woods alive with game. The fertile ground was supposed to be excellent for farming. The area had recently been opened for homesteading, and many people had come up from the States to give it a try.

These people had cleared fields from virgin forests, and they were living in houses they had built with the logs. The Territory was building a road to Seward, and a few trucks were starting to use it. They were also building roads to Homer and Anchorage. Predictions were that in five years, Kenai would be a very busy place. The airfield was excellent, and it had a reputation for more good flying days a year than any other airfield in Alaska.

About 15 miles up the river I found my dream homestead. Standing on a bluff, I could look out across the river flowing in its fertile valley down to the sparkling water of Cook Inlet, with the ethereal snow-capped peaks beyond. Nothing could have been more beautiful. The idea of homesteading hit most of us on the ship like a virulent disease. We were all out looking for land. When we returned and sat around eating the fine turkey dinner that Ed had prepared, we compared notes. Amazingly, we had all picked the same location.

When we slid out of the river into Cook Inlet, we found wicked-looking waves, and the captain headed for Seldovia and Mrs. Anderson's dock. She greeted us, and then as the wind picked up, she once again asked us to move to the middle of the bay, afraid that the force of the wind on the ship would pull down her dock. It appeared that we were getting out of Cook Inlet this year just in time.

The next morning Dr. Swanson received a wire from Dr. Albrecht in Juneau, giving him permission to leave the ship to return to his expectant wife. He caught a plane to Anchorage and then to Juneau. Our staff and crew were rapidly disappearing. Tatitlek was the only town left on the schedule, so Dr. Swanson gave Kitty and me instructions on what to do there.

Captain Kippola decided to stay in Seldovia another day because of the poor weather. Some of the crew members were annoyed because he refused to lower the boat, claiming he was holding them prisoners on the ship. More probably he was wary of losing more crew members. I wanted to X-ray the people of Seldovia, but Dr. Swanson had expected we would leave that afternoon and did not think there would be enough time. So I painted the lab while Kitty and Peggy worked on records. Dr. Pope extracted the broken tooth of a Seldovian citizen who had come out to the ship in his own boat. Harry Halvorsen, a personable young man, came on as the new deckhand.

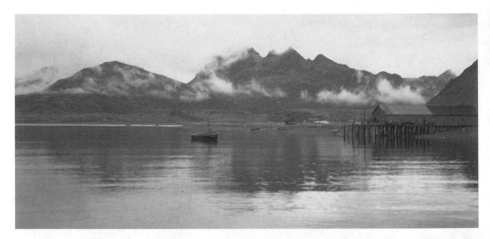

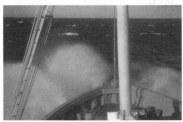

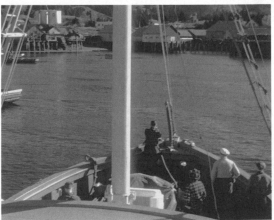

Top: Old Harbor.
Middle: left, rough weather in
Cook Inlet; *right,* coming into
Seldovia.
Bottom: Columbia Glacier.

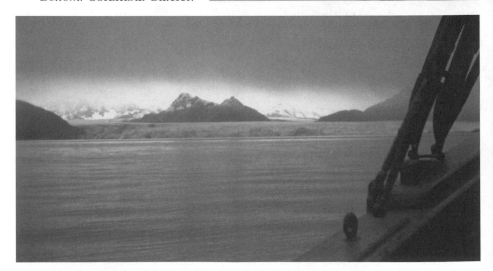

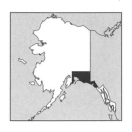

Prince William Sound and Gulf of Alaska

Seward
Thursday, October 16, to Friday, October 17

In Seward, the first thing Kitty and I did was to look for Mrs. Arave, the territorial nurse who was our contact for mail there. But she no longer lived at the address we had, and her name was not in the phone book. So we had no mail—an all-too-familiar pattern. Soon most of the ship's complement had scattered to the various bars and the movies. I enjoyed window shopping—just looking at different things was fun.

The next morning Kitty, the Popes, and I hurried out to the Home in the Woods TB sanitarium to collect the dental supplies they had put aside for Dr. Pope. We were happy to see that Dr. Valle, the doctor who was so enthusiastic on our last visit, was still there. He had found an anesthesiologist and was doing thoracoplasties. That meant he collapsed a portion of a tuberculous lung by removing some ribs, thus giving the diseased tissue a chance to rest and heal.

When we arrived he was in the midst of a bronchoscopy (inserting a long hollow tube with a light on the end into the bronchial tubes to look around). He invited us to stay and watch, arranging the operation so we could see what he was doing. He explained everything he did and why he did it, even letting us look down the tube to see what he was seeing. His employees worshipped him, and we could see why.

Later we found that no one there had been paid anything but board and room for the last eight weeks. The staff stayed on because Dr. Valle was so enthusiastic and believed so much in what he was doing. Kitty and I benefited from talking to him. We could, with much greater conviction, tell discouraged villagers that indeed, the most modern treatments were being used in Alaska. Dr. Valle in turn quizzed us about the types and extent of TB cases we had found.

While we were talking after the operation, one of the fellows working there came up and handed Dr. Valle an Anchorage paper. Large black headlines shouted, "Seward Sanitarium to Close in One Month."

Dr. Valle looked at it, and laughed, "What, again! The papers have been saying we are going to close for the last three or four months, and we are still going strong. I just heard yesterday they found a source of money to pay us." Greatly encouraged and cheered by this remarkable man, we returned to the *Hygiene*.

Just before we left for Chenega, the missing Mrs. Arave arrived with a box of mail sent air express. Kitty explained, "We tried to find you but no one at that address knew you."

The nurse laughed, "I'm not surprised. I've recently married, changed my name, and moved."

Good news from my mother and a long letter from the handsome young schoolteacher on Sanak Island lifted my spirits. I had wondered if Dick's and my paths would ever cross again.

Just before we took off, a telegram arrived from the Juneau office adding Chenega and Ellamar to our scheduled stop at Tatitlek. Dr. Armstrong and Mrs. Lindley from Valdez would work with us.

Chenega
Saturday, October 18

It was strange not having Dr. Swanson, but the work went well. We referred several emergency medical cases that came to us to the doctors at Valdez or Cordova. The people in Prince William Sound were not nearly as isolated as those on the Alaska Peninsula or on the Bering Sea. They were only one day away from medical help, and Mrs. Lindley could get to them for follow-up work. We were taking the X-rays to Juneau, where a TB specialist would read them. Without a doctor, we had to limit our X-ray program to small survey X-rays, except on cases that had been positive the year before. We could still perform immunizations, blood tests, a sanitary survey, prenatal conferences, and movies in each town. Kitty and I both thought we could have done more.

I complained to Kitty, "I've seen enough X-rays to readily recognize any obvious abnormalities; it's stupid to be here and not take a large X-ray when the small film is abnormal. That doesn't mean I am going to take over diagnosing a disease, but at least the doctor who is reading the abnormal X-ray will have the material to work with. I may miss some of the finer points, but this way we are missing all of them."

Kitty sympathized and said, "I could do child health conferences but I didn't know we were going to make these extra stops, so I didn't think to establish standing orders for the treatment of scabies."

The whole concept seemed ridiculous to me. Kitty had been treating scabies since we started, and now, even though scabies was a problem, she couldn't do anything about it. She didn't feel it was imperative, since Mrs.

Lindley expected to visit the village later. I had become aware that many nurses were strongly indoctrinated to having doctor's orders for every move. Maybe this was necessary in the States, but it seemed out of place under the conditions we were experiencing.

Chenega was the town where I had purchased my baidarka with so much enthusiasm the previous year. I asked Mr. Poling if he thought any of the Natives might buy it back, explaining how much more comfortable the kayak was. He said, "I'll be glad to return the $40 you paid for it." That limited my equipment on board ship to one kayak, one bicycle, one pair of skis, and one set of reindeer horns. The horns, secured to the top of the mast, made it easy to spot the *Hygiene* from a distance. I thought they added character as well.

Tatitlek
Sunday, October 19, to Monday, October 20

On the way to Tatitlek, Kitty and Gus had a furious argument about sleeping accommodations for the visiting doctor and nurse. The plan was for Kitty and Mrs. Lindley, the visiting nurse, to use Dr. Swanson's now-empty stateroom and give Kitty's stateroom to the visiting doctor. While Kitty cleaned her quarters for Dr. Armstrong, Gus insisted that the assistant engineer should have her room, and the visiting doctor should sleep in the fo'c'sle. At this point the pair were having a lot of ups and many downs in their romance. The captain settled the sleeping arrangements following the original plan.

The first snow of the year fell on the *Hygiene* as we traveled. It was a gentle snowfall, but it brought back vivid memories of the icing problems of the year before.

Dr. Armstrong and Mrs. Lindley, the Valdez nurse, sent word that they would not be at Tatitlek until Monday. Rather than lose time, Kitty and I proceeded to X-ray, immunize, and run blood tests in the village. Kitty showed movies in the evening. We were cheerfully working on Sunday because of the time lost due to bad weather. For some reason, much of the crew's tension and stubbornness about Sunday work had left with Dr. Swanson.

Mrs. Lindley arrived on Jim Dolan's boat the next morning with the news that Dr. Armstrong had had a heart attack the night before. She went ashore for conferences with the patients who had outstanding health problems. Since no other transportation was available, she requested that we take her back to Valdez.

Kitty inaugurated her set of prenatal Kodachrome slides on all the women and some teenagers. She felt they conveyed the ideas she was trying to express, and hoped the visual impact would reach the midwife, who was hard of hearing and who practiced bleeding to relieve the aches and pains of her patients. Kitty made a point of inviting the midwife's daughter, one of the best volunteer workers, to the class. She hoped the girl would influence her mother to better midwifery methods. We doubted that we could have secured a chest X-ray of the midwife without the daughter's help.

Valdez
Tuesday, October 21

When we returned Mrs. Lindley to Valdez, we visited Dr. Armstrong. This remarkable man, hospitalized with a heart attack, was trying to supervise the care of a possible Cesarean section. He insisted that we brief him on conditions we had found in Prince William Sound. After a short visit to Mrs. Lindley's comfortable home, I returned to the ship with little desire to trade my stateroom and exciting life for a cozy and tranquil home ashore. While we were gone, Dr. Pope had been besieged with patients who wanted him to start a practice in Valdez.

Cordova
Wednesday, October 22, to Friday, October 31

At last we completed all of our assignments, and we headed for Juneau, with a stop in Cordova for fuel. There Captain Kippola decided to wait until noon the following day after he listened to the latest weather forecast. The prediction was for hurricane-force winds to hit the Gulf that night.

As long as we were there, Mrs. Hodge, the local nurse, wanted us to do an X-ray survey of the town. We told her Cordova was not on our schedule because the highway unit would be along soon to do that. Mrs. Hodge asked us to at least X-ray the school children, explaining that we were there, but many obstacles might prevent the mobile unit from getting to Cordova at that time of year. We agreed with her but explained we could not go ahead without orders from Juneau. So she wired Dr. Albrecht requesting that the children be X-rayed. She would have included everyone, but Dr. Pope vetoed that. He wanted nothing to delay our return.

Pending an answer, Kitty and I went ahead with the plans, so we could make the most of the three hours the next morning. The school principal and newspaper editor helped spread the word.

Promptly at 9:30 a.m. the first children arrived. We had not received an answer to our telegram, so my team and I decided to start X-raying. We took 194 X-rays in two and one-half hours. It was a truly cooperative effort. Mrs. Hodge changed film in the dark room, Peggy took chest measurements, I took the X-rays and changed the cassettes, while Kitty positioned the patients and changed the numbers. Everyone pitched in with a will, and we had a great time working as a team. When we were nearly through, a reply to the previous day's telegram came from Dr. Swanson telling us, "Do not X-ray the school children. Take large films on last year's cases." Since we had essentially completed the job, we went ahead and finished.

In the meantime, the captain had received a weather report saying that the hurricane was raging in the Gulf. That meant we would lay over at least another day. Mrs. Hodge rounded up as many of last year's positive cases as she could find, and we took the large films that afternoon. It was so frustrating to just sit there knowing we could have X-rayed the whole town while we waited. The townspeople didn't understand and neither did we, so we worked on reports and inventories.

The storm raged for two more days. Our shipmates who had not crossed the Gulf of Alaska the previous winter had no concept of the relief and joy we felt at being firmly and securely tied to a sheltered dock. The hurricane made the headlines. Finally even the Popes stopped pushing the captain to leave.

For once we were getting our fill of movies. Our crew had often wished we could carry films for our own entertainment as the Coast Guard ships did. We were all sick of "Good-bye Mr. Germ," "It Can Be Done," and the other health films.

On Saturday morning, with Dr. Pope egging him on, Captain Kippola decided to take the *Hygiene* out to look at the Gulf even though the weather reports were still bad. After bouncing around for a couple of hours, we returned to Port Etches, a protected small bay on Hinchinbrook Island. The wind howled and the wind blew the rain parallel to the water in great quantities. Kitty, Gus, and I were completely happy with the captain's decision to wait for better weather. The dentist and his wife were perturbed by the arrangement, but they had been perturbed with everything, so it didn't worry anyone very much.

We passed the time reading, knitting, or playing cards, and we had some rousing games of ping pong on the salon table. The ping pong games were rather different from the usual type in that an inch-high lip surrounded the table. The table was shorter and wider than standard, and only three feet separated it from the benches running around the walls of the salon. The technique was to make the ball hit the table lip at just the right angle so it would be impossible to return. I had become proficient at that maneuver.

On Monday, Dr. Pope again urged Captain Kippola to take the *Hygiene* out into the Gulf. Huge waves battered us, and the conditions were worse than they had been on Saturday. There seemed no end to the storm. At last Dr. Pope accepted the situation and busied himself building cupboards in his office.

I went into the salon Monday night, saying, "I've finished knitting my socks, I've read all the books, answered all my letters, and brought my diary up to date. I hope we get out of here pretty soon, but understand, I'm not complaining, just stating the facts." Ed worried that he would run out of food in a few more days. Then the ship truly would be an unhappy place.

Kitty wrote a long list of recommendations for the future and caught up on her reports that she was supposed to write in an "objective manner."

"How can I write objectively when we are all so close and everything anyone does affects the rest of us?" she asked. "It would be like ignoring the subconscious in studying a psychiatric problem."

On Tuesday, Kitty and I took buckets of soapy water and cleaned the entire clinic with scrub brushes. The rest of the crew razzed us, saying, "The Gulf will have huge waves when we cross it and the salt water will leak all over what you have just done." But we went ahead, figuring the weather would have to improve. Besides, it felt good to be doing something. I was so thankful to have a friend like Kitty on board. She stayed on an even keel and was easy to get along with. She always thought of things to do to help other people and was a truly unselfish person.

While we were scrubbing, we discussed our thoughts on the overall program. I was usually the optimist on board. Since we had worked in the Yukon Delta, however, and especially since the return visits to the Alaska Peninsula and Kodiak Island, I had felt overwhelmed and depressed at the magnitude of the job we were trying to do. The problems we had to overcome were so varied and seemed uncontrollable. The unpredictable and violent weather of the Yukon Delta area, with its vast expanses of shallow water and mud flats on the sea side and miles of marsh on the land side, made it impossible to plan any kind of scheduled program. Planes were the only dependable access, and they could not be that predictable. Even if equipment could be flown into these isolated villages, where would the people running it stay? Where could they sleep and eat?

Then, assuming that hospital beds were available, how would the people be transported to them? Families would be separated for years. The patient, often a child, might well be transported to a hospital where no one spoke or understood his language. Of course, that was better than having him spread the disease and die.

The problem of staffing was obvious. Very few people wanted to work under the stressful conditions involved. This was true of all the ship's personnel, from deckhand to doctor. The constant changeover of medical personnel and crew added to the difficulties. Kitty, Gus, and I were the only three who had accepted the rigors of the work and life on board ship for even one year. We did not stay in a job like that for the money. It required a dedication to the people we were trying to help.

Money was another problem; the crew and staff on the ship felt a need to pinch every penny. The Department of Health was trying to stretch every dollar, so they sent the ship out with an inadequate number of men, especially when we were in the Bering Sea. For safety the ship should have had three crewmen for each job and two dories, each with a spare motor, as well as adequate water tanks. Part of the problem was ignorance of the conditions we would encounter.

But the greatest need was to treat some of the cases we had discovered before the villagers became totally disillusioned and refused to cooperate with the program. Basically the problem lay in trying to serve a wide variety of cultures. These varied from traditional, non-English-speaking, totally isolated communities in the Bering Sea to modern towns with airports and all the accouterments of the civilization of the 1940s. Dr. Albrecht and many of the lawmakers fought desperately for money to make the program feasible. The Department of Health had a great deal of catching up to do, but so did all the other agencies of the Alaskan government. Alaska had been ignored too long.

We discussed all this while waiting for the hurricane to end, and we realized that weather had to be one of our worst problems in making any kind of plans.

Later in the afternoon the Coast Guard Cutter *Analga* slipped into the sheltered anchorage. They told Captain Kippola he had done the right thing by staying in a protected location. The storm had been long and violent.

Kitty showed all her slides on Tuesday night. Everyone except the three crew members last hired had seen them, but it was a change from card-playing and complaining. Even Gus looked at the familiar pictures without grumbling. Kitty, elated, told me, "Maybe Gus and I do have some of the same interests after all. I've been worried about that."

Wednesday morning dawned bright and calm. The weather report was good. At 9 a.m. we left for Juneau and did not have to turn back. The trip across the gulf was smooth, with a full moon both nights. We arrived in Juneau at 8:30 a.m. on the morning of October 31, 11 days after we had first tried to leave Cordova, and four months and 22 days after our departure for the Bering Sea. Four of the original group were still aboard.

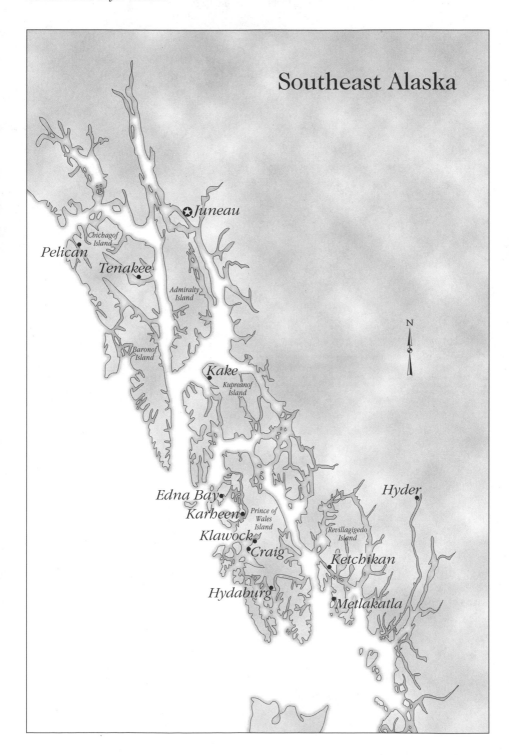

Southeast Alaska

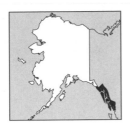

6

Good-Bye

Juneau to Hydaburg and Kake
Friday, Oct 31 to Monday, November 24

AFTER TEN DAYS OF VACATION and resupply in Juneau, we were on the way again. Our mission: to put up exhibits for the Alaska Native Brotherhood Convention in Hydaburg. The brotherhood was formed of all the aboriginal Natives in Southeast Alaska. Each village had sent from three to five delegates, for a total of nearly 100.

The Indians, excellent extemporaneous speakers, had a delightful sense of humor. Their poise, quick wit, and intelligence constantly impressed us. The difference in sophistication among the Indians of Southeast Alaska and some of the Eskimos and Aleuts we had seen so recently was tremendous. The northern Natives, while not familiar with modern technology, were very sophisticated in dealing with the problems they faced in the severe climate and remoteness of the areas where they lived. No wonder the Alaska legislature had problems enacting laws that would care for and be fair to all. It was worse when the Congress in Washington, D.C., with little or no knowledge of the varied cultures and conditions it was trying to improve, enacted those laws.

Dr. McMinimy, the TB consultant in Juneau, a slightly pudgy but affable man, would be our doctor for the next month. Dr. Pope remained as dentist. In addition, Maggie Bogue, assistant nursing supervisor, and Ralph Williams, Director of

Laboratories, came along. Our doctors gave their speeches, the nurses set up demonstrations and showed movies, and I showed those who were interested what the TB germ looked like under the microscope. The Brotherhood listened attentively to our talks and demonstrations, but they raked the people from the Bureau of Indian Affairs over the coals.

They raised one question that applied to us concerning racial discrimination. One of the Native speakers showed a concern that statistics on tuberculosis in Alaska were expressed by race. He believed this might lead or was leading toward discriminatory remarks and practices against the Natives of Alaska.

Dr. McMinimy assured the delegate that the Territorial Department of Health had no intention of showing discrimination. He attempted to show the convention that statistics on tuberculosis were extremely important in order to get an accurate picture of the problem for better combating the disease—for example, to provide hospital beds in locations that would best serve the various groups.

After we left Hydaburg for Kake, the ship's heating system broke down, and the only warm places were the engine room, the galley, and our beds. We ran in to Petersburg, the closest town where we could get a heater. After it was installed, the dining salon became another warm oasis.

The program at Kake went smoothly and quickly because we had been there in February. We checked the positive cases, and the doctor and Kitty held the usual clinics and conferences.

Our timing was good, and we returned to Juneau the day before Thanksgiving and spent the holiday eating a fine dinner that Ed Stice, the bo's'n, had prepared for us. It is difficult to explain the bonds of friendship that existed among those of us who had been on board together. It had nothing to do with romance and wasn't even a family feeling, because our paths went in completely different directions when we were ashore, except that Kitty's and Gus's lives had of late merged more. The general bond was more of a special consideration for each other's feelings, and when this was present, we had a happy ship, no matter what the surrounding weather or work circumstances might be.

Juneau to Pelican
Tuesday, November 25, to Saturday, December 13

In Juneau Dr. Hazel Blair came aboard as ship's physician. She was about my age, dark-haired and attractive in a gentle, quiet way. She made a good first impression that grew even better in the 10 days we worked at Pelican, a town that appeared to be built on stilts. Our program ran smoothly. Kitty and Gus were spending more and more time on walks, and their conversations seemed to stop when others were present. Rumor and gossip were circulating around the ship. I was sure they would tell us the news when there was some.

Tenakee
Saturday, December 13, to Friday, December 19

We sailed smoothly to Tenakee, a far better situation than the embattled, ice-laden voyage of the previous year. On our arrival we trekked up the hillside and picked greens to decorate the ship for Christmas. After everything was in place and the tree trimmed, Kitty and Gus put an end to the rumors and suspense. They planned to be married December 23. We were not surprised, even though they had had their share of stormy times. It had been a discreet romance, which was remarkable under the close conditions in which we lived and worked. All who could went up to the ice-cream parlor and bought ice-cream cones to celebrate.

The next day the happy couple came down to the lab for the blood tests they needed to get their marriage license. I drew blood from Kitty with no problem. Then Gus came in and sat down. He took one look at the syringe and needle and before I even put the tourniquet around his arm, he fainted. After he came to, he decided to wait and have me do it the next day. This time we blindfolded him and Kitty held his hand, but when he felt the tourniquet around his arm, he became white and woozy. We began to wonder if they would be able to get married after all. Dr. Blair suggested he lie on the examining table. I dispensed with the tourniquet and while Kitty diverted his attention, I slipped the needle in his vein and drew some blood.

Juneau
Friday, December 19, to Sunday, December 21

Earlier I had made a reservation on the steamer to Seattle for December 21 and was unable to be at Kitty and Gus's wedding, which was a great disappointment. I gave a dinner for them and our friends at the Baranof Hotel, and they all took me to the steamer afterward.

What a surprise to find Kitty and Gus, Mr. and Mrs. Angus Gair, waiting on the dock in Seattle when the steamer pulled in on Christmas Eve. Radiantly happy, they showed me their apartment and told me about their wedding and their plans for the next month. They were two grand people.

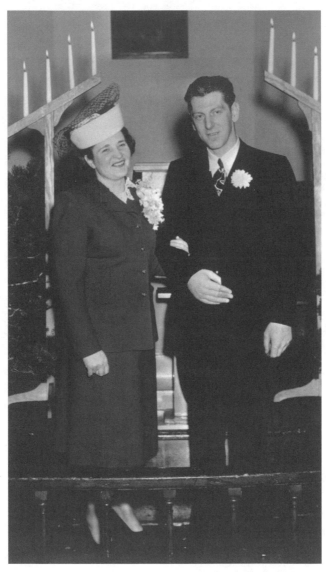

Mr. and Mrs. Angus Gair,
wedding picture, Christmas, 1948

During my Christmas vacation in Seattle it was obvious that my mother needed me and that I could no longer stay on the Hygiene with a clear conscience. My brother could stay with her until spring, and then he would have to leave. As much as I enjoyed the work and life on board ship, I knew it would not be right for me to take off on another trip to the far north. Sadly I told Dr. Albrecht I would have to resign in the spring. He suggested that I take a year's leave of absence. The thought that I could return made it a bit easier to leave this life I loved. While the next few months were not tremendously exciting or different from the stops we had made the year before, I treasured every experience and relationship, knowing it would soon come to an end.

1948

Craig and Klawock
Saturday, January 10, to Tuesday, February 3

Maggie Bogue, who filled in for Kitty, had been on the little *Hy-Gene* that had made the original small-scale survey of TB in Southeast Alaska. Thoroughly familiar with every aspect of the Department of Health, she had lived in most of the towns and villages for varying periods of time and knew the people and their problems. Dr. Blair enjoyed her assurance, calmness, and sense of humor as much as I did, and our work in Craig went smoothly. A highlight in my life at that time was a letter and Christmas package from my friend Dick on Sanak Island. That seemed so long ago. I was delighted that he had remembered me.

After we moved to Klawock, we again had to cope with a balky X-ray machine. I could not put my finger on a specific problem. One morning the generator wouldn't start. I said it missed Gus. When it eventually roared to life, the X-rays were poor. Then for a time the X-rays were excellent. The generator started to hiccup. Again poor X-rays. At least we were someplace where we could communicate. Finally we received a message from Juneau to proceed to Ketchikan. Mr. Martinson would meet us there, as would Kitty and Gus.

Ketchikan
Wednesday, February 4, to Thursday, February 19

We spent 15 frustrating days in Ketchikan. The generator seemed to recover, and again we joked that it had missed Gus. Marty concentrated his efforts on the X-ray machine. It would take beautiful pictures, and just when he was wiping his hands and getting ready to fly back to Seattle, they became terrible again. When he was sure the X-ray machine was behaving, the generator would not start, even with Gus there to give it a friendly kick. The weather was extremely cold, and the men nearly froze their fingers working on the generator out on the deck. As the days passed, we seesawed between hope and despair.

Marty kept saying, as he paced up and down the deck. "I smell a rat." I thought it was a figure of speech and that he meant someone might be deliberately doing something to the machine. It turned out he meant it literally.

The generator was in two sections, and the trouble seemed to be in the part with the motor. One day Gus opened the other side to check something and saw some scraps of paper. Further investigation revealed a rat's nest. After the men poked around some more they found an electrocuted rat lying across two wires. It was delicately balanced and with the motion of the boat it sometimes caused a short circuit and sometimes did not. I was relieved that this episode had occurred where we could get help, and not in the Bering Sea.

Edna Bay and Karheen
Friday, February 20, to Tuesday, February 24

With the X-ray machine and generator again their dependable selves, we left for Edna Bay, a lumber camp of about 60 loggers, and its branch camp at Karheen with 20 men. Our work was so easy where everyone was relatively healthy and spoke English. We learned that away from the main camp the men lived in wanigans, houses built on rafts that could be moved and tied to shore near the areas to be logged.

One evening the camp superintendent offered to take us abalone hunting because the tide would be at minus two feet. We climbed onto his humdurgen, a small sturdy workboat. The abalones were supposed to grow best where the open ocean acted on them. So we went out of the sheltered waters to a reef at the mouth of the inlet that was bare at this tide. The humdurgen stayed in deep water, and a skiff deposited us on a pile of rocks covered with kelp and slippery seaweed only about a foot above water level. A good swell was running, and the waves would come crashing around

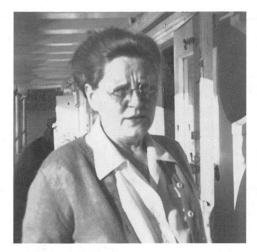
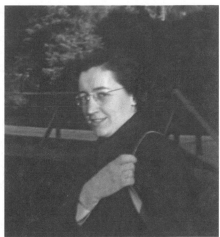

Top: left, Maggie;
right, Dr. Blair.
Middle: Gus and Mr.
Brown.
Bottom: Rex and Mr.
Brown, bellies.

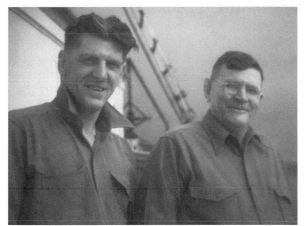

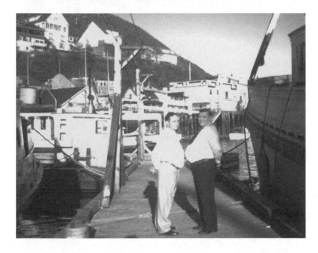

the rocks and sometimes over our feet. A full moon gave eerie light when we started, but then a snow squall obscured it, and our flashlights were terribly puny as we stumbled around in the slippery darkness, water periodically washing over our feet while we pried off the stubborn abalones with tire irons. I was relieved when someone decided the tide was coming in, and we had better get out of there.

Most of us had never eaten abalone before. We found that it was almost as hard to prepare them as to harvest them. They reminded me of a piece of old tire, but after we had beaten them to a pulp and ground them they had a delicious flavor.

Klawock (continued)
Wednesday, February 25, to Monday, March 15

We returned to finish the work in Klawock that had been cut short by the balky generator. Saturday morning Mr. and Mrs. Stenson, the teachers, came and told us in great excitement that the herring were spawning on Fish Egg Island. They invited us to join their group, to bring a picnic lunch and some butter, and to be ready at noon. We didn't know why this was a cause for excitement, but we were willing to find out. At noon they picked us up with a fishing boat and took us to a protected small bay about an hour's run from town. There they ferried us, laden with our picnic baskets, to shore where we built a bonfire. This time we were not alone. It was a beautiful day, and most of the villagers were there, their bonfires strung around the crescent bay like a necklace. The larger boats were anchored in the entrance.

Two days previously, the men had cut hemlock boughs and tied them to floats anchored over the surface of the bay. Now they were harvesting their crop. The herring laid their eggs on the branches and needles until they became almost completely white. They reminded me of large clusters of mistletoe. Each family had its stack of egg-covered branches, a big fire with a kettle of boiling water, and another of hot seal oil. Flocks of happy children played on the shore. A holiday atmosphere prevailed as the women visited, and the men joked and told stories.

All afternoon everyone guzzled herring eggs. The Indians gave us a stack of egg-covered branches and showed us how to dip a branch in the boiling water for about 20 seconds, then in the hot seal oil. (We were glad we had been warned to bring butter.) They would then strip the eggs from the needles between their teeth—a knack I had trouble learning. I kept getting the needles, too.

Herring darted about in the bay that was milky with all the eggs. The sea lions came to feed on them, and we saw herds of these large beasts jumping clear of the water. The seagulls were also in on the act, so many they looked like a white cloud. Five bald eagles soared above them.

Craig
Tuesday, March 16 to Wednesday, March 24

We returned to Craig to continue our program of X-rays and clinics. One of the active cases we found was the school janitor. The townspeople quickly organized a benefit dance to raise money to help him take his family of four children back to their home state of California where he hoped he could be hospitalized sooner than in Alaska. He also had relatives there to help his family. The many bars generously donated whiskey for the occasion and when the proceeds from the dance and bars were totaled they amounted to $876 in the one night. The churches collected $60 and gave his wife a personal shower. It was heartwarming to see how the town pitched in to help an unfortunate victim of this miserable disease. I wished the same sort of thing could be done for the multitude of helpless Natives who had to hunt and fish and who were spreading their illness to others while waiting without hope for the hospital beds that had been needed for so long.

Hydaburg and vicinity
Wednesday, March 24, to Thursday, April 8

We moved to Hydaburg just before Easter weekend. On Good Friday after dinner, Kitty and I decided to color Easter eggs. As usual, our activities were greeted with barely tolerant amusement. After we boiled a bunch of eggs and were dyeing them, the fellows began to give us advice. Kitty managed to get an egg in Gus's hand when he started to tell her how to draw a face. "Show me," she said. Gradually, one by one each crew member became involved until we were all sitting around the table with an egg or two. Once they started, the fellows became enthusiastic—no simple colored eggs for them. They made geometric designs, clowns, several ladies with hair and fancy hats, and even a couple of caricatures of people on the ship. The evening was hilarious, and the picture of those rough, tough seamen with their big clumsy hands decorating hats to put on eggs is one I'll never forget.

Fred Mueller, who had come aboard in Kodiak, left us, and Rex, who had left the year before, rejoined the ship. It was good to have him back.

From April 8 to April 11 we worked at small, mostly white logging camps and quarries. These were View Cove, Deer Bay, Sulzer, and Nutkwa. The scenery had been particularly spectacular the last ten days. When we reached Ketchikan, where we laid over from April 12 to 15, we realized why. It had not rained. We had been blessed with blue skies and sunshine throughout that time. The drought was the main topic of conversation. Everyone we talked to complained about the heat and dust. They worried because the water supply was getting low.

Sorrowfully I made my reservation on the steamer for Seattle for May 10.

Hyder
Friday, April 16, to Tuesday, April 20

We sailed south to the border between Canada and Alaska and headed up Portland Canal. For 90 spectacular miles this fjord cut through 8000- to 9000-foot peaks that soared skyward from the mile-wide channel. As we penetrated this cleft in the mountains, the snow line came closer and closer to the water until the two merged. When we reached Hyder, almost a ghost town with a population of 35 (we had expected 100), the ground was covered with three feet of snow even though it was mid-April.

The many disintegrating, windowless buildings resting precariously on rickety, worm-eaten pilings were evidence of great activity in the past. The dock looked equally unsafe, and we obtained permission from the Canadian officials to tie up to a more substantial structure on their side of the canal in the town of Stewart. It, too, looked deserted, although 200 to 300 people were living in the area.These towns were ports for the large gold mines in the mountains behind them.

Dr. Blair and Kitty spent the morning looking for people to X-ray, and I took a total of 15. In the afternoon, the commissioner took us up to Canada's Premier Gold Mine. Riding in a big old bus, we climbed on a narrow road to an elevation of 3000 feet in 17 miles. The snow was piled eight to 10 feet high on each side of the road, and some of the switchbacks were so sharp we had to back up to get around them. It was raining when we started, but soon we were plowing through a blizzard. Our driver described the processes used to extract and concentrate the gold, silver, and lead. These concentrates were carried to the dock on an aerial tramway that returned to the mine carrying the fuel they used. The mine had been in operation about 30 years and had produced $20 million in profits.

About 200 people lived at the mine, where a swimming pool, tennis and badminton courts, movies, stores, and a hospital helped them cope with their isolation. Our work was completed, and we headed back to Ketchikan to pick up my replacement. I was to spend the next 10 days teaching her my job.

The trip to Hyder completed the mission we had started two years earlier: "Survey the coastal population of Alaska to determine the incidence of tuberculosis." This we had done from the Bering Sea to the Canadian border. That simple-sounding directive gave no indication of the immensity and complexity of the undertaking. It was one thing to know where TB was prevalent, but so many other factors were involved—transportation, separation of family members for years, language, other diverse medical problems, education, and sufficient hospital beds with staff to care for the patients. It had not been possible to limit our work to "just" a survey for TB.

The results of the survey bore out what had been suspected concerning the disease's prevalence and distribution. The areas with high rates of infection were far worse, however, than anyone had estimated. Tuberculosis, normally an endemic disease, had reached epidemic proportions and threatened to wipe out some villages unless we could change its course.

We who had been on the ship for two years had learned a great deal about human relationships, both with the Natives we served, and with each other. When I remembered the discouragement I felt at the end of the Bering Sea trip, I realized that all of us, crew and staff, had done a tremendous job. Sometimes we wondered if we had made a difference. Time gave me the perspective that we had to meet the challenges one step at a time, and we had made a good first step. The full expansion of Dr. Albrecht's aggressive program on increased tuberculosis control, along with the use of BCG in certain isolated areas and the development of the drug isonazid, virtually wiped tuberculosis out as a major killer. I hope this book will bring to life the daily struggles of the heroic nurses and doctors as well as the teachers, missionaries, and bush pilots who took part in this fight against an epidemic-scale disease, and that it will give hope to those caught in future outbreaks of diseases that might occur. I was happy to have had a small part in this achievement.

Metlakatla and Ketchikan
Wednesday, April 21, to Monday, May 10

My last few weeks were busy training my replacement as we went through our familiar routines in Metlakatla. Every day seemed to pass more swiftly, and I dreaded the final good-byes. My friends and shipmates did so much to help and cheer me that last week. I couldn't keep the tears back when they had a farewell dinner and presented me with a camera to replace the one I had dropped overboard shortly before. When I sadly climbed on the *Aleutian* bound for Seattle, the whole bunch was there shouting, "See you next year!"

But, when the year had gone by, I had to send in my resignation because I was still needed at home. I had an interesting job at the newly opened medical school at the University of Washington, and it led to marriage and a family of my own.

As the years passed, and I lived in Seattle, surrounded by walls and thousands of people, cars, roads, and traffic jams, my Alaska experiences would occasionally spring vividly to life. For a short time I would leave prosaic, middle-class America to revisit that Alaska unknown to so many. My mind would go to that other world in the north, not the tourist show, but the place where one had to search to find a small village in the huge emptiness of the tundra and the sea; the small community dominated by its priest, church, and smoking mountain; the articulate, intelligent Natives discussing their people's problems, and the joy on the face of an old woman over a card saying "TB-neg." I wonder, is it still there?

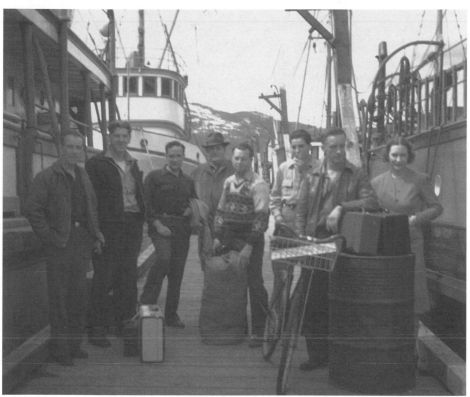

Good-bye

Epilogue 1997

THE *HYGIENE* AND other health ships ceased operations in 1952 due to drastic cuts in federal funding. The Territorial Health Department faced a dilemma; not only were finances a problem, but it would be difficult to find medical team personnel willing to live an itinerant life based on carrying all their equipment and food as well as sleeping bags, often by dog team, bush plane, or small boat, to primitive villages. However the itinerant Public Health Nurses met the challenge and formed the backbone of the public health delivery system at the village level, which is still in place and will continue to have a role in the search for and control of tuberculosis into the twenty-first century.

In the last 50 years, many changes in Alaska have greatly improved the delivery of health care. In 1959 Alaska became a state, and Alaskans took charge of their own destiny. Transportation and communication improved dramatically. The State of Alaska established an excellent marine highway system to serve its widespread coastal population, enabling patients to reach medical treatment and vice versa.

The Alaska Native Claims Settlement Act of 1971 (amended 1986) awarded money and land to the 13 Native Corporations. The act established a framework by which Native Associations could, among other things, assume ownership and development of their land and gradually take responsibility for developing, operating or refining their own health services.

A Community Health Aide (CHA) program, which began as an unpaid volunteer-interpreter and doctor-nurse helper system in the villages, was formalized into an organized training program that led to paid employment. Today there are CHAs working in every Native village of any size.

Through the use of satellites and Alaska's outstanding telecommunication system, it is possible for trained CHAs in the most remote villages to access highly sophisticated equipment, and to talk to and exchange medical information such as X-rays and EKGs, with doctors in the medical centers of the larger cities. All these factors, combined with the dramatic change in treatment of tuberculosis after the discovery of effective chemotherapy, replaced years of hospitalization, which often resulted in broken families and poor morale, with a six-month course of home medication.

In 1948 Alaska's population of 81,445 had an estimated 4000 active cases of tuberculosis. Fifty percent of the population had been X-rayed, and 2270 cases were on record. A 1981 report by Robert Fraser, Chief of Alaska's Section of Communicable Disease Control, states that 32 years later, in 1980, a population of 400,481 showed only 76 cases.

A communication from Dr. Michael Jones, formerly in the Division of Public Health, Section of Epidemiology, states that the former director of Alaska's Tuberculosis Control Program believes that

> While TB rates have dropped dramatically in Alaska, and the prevalence of the disease among younger individuals is quite low, the disease still remains difficult to control in the Native population because so many were infected at the time when effective preventive treatment was not yet available. In the 1940s and early 1950s, for instance, the *infection* rate—not the incidence rate of active tuberculosis disease—was nearly 100% among Yupik Eskimos by late adolescence or early adulthood. This large pool of infected persons, many of whom did not receive an adequate course of isonazid still, 40 to 50 years later, have some risk of developing the disease and transmitting it to others. Infected immigrants from TB-epidemic areas (example Southeast Asia) add to the pool.

Meanwhile this germ can be as deadly as ever, because a new strain that is resistant to the drugs which brought it under control has developed. So Alaska's search for this killer goes on.

Did we make a difference? We believe so. We penetrated some of Alaska's remotest areas in our search for the hot spots of the tuberculosis epidemic. We, along with the heroic public health nurses and doctors, school teachers, and missionaries, were among those at the leading edge in educating the residents on how to improve their health.

Kitty and Gus remained on the *Hygiene* until it went out of service. Kitty earned an M.A. degree in Child Psychiatric Nursing at Boston University and then worked for the school system in Juneau until she retired in 1971. During those years she was actively involved in the Alaska Nurses Association, edited The Alaska Nurse and was on several hospital boards and the Hospice board in Juneau. Kitty now lives in Wasilla, Alaska, near her son and grandson. After he left the *Hygiene,* Gus worked as an engineer for the Alaska Marine Highway System until he retired in 1971. He died in 1977.

Dr. Schwinge served in various positions in Alaska until 1959, when she returned to the East Coast. She spent three years at the U.S.P.H.S. Hospital in Lexington, KY, specializing in psychiatry, and continues to practice in New York and Pennsylvania. She married Gino Ruggiero in 1961, and they raised twin sons.

Susie (Susan Hull Meredith) and her husband Jim retired to a log cabin, which they built on San Juan Island in the State of Washington. There Susie keeps a fiberglass version of her Eskimo kayak on the beach and paddles whenever she can.

After the Hygiene was retired, she was converted to a yacht and named the Westwind. We have not been able to find out what happened to her. We would like to hear from anyone who knows her fate and from any crew members or their families who worked on the *Hygiene,* the *Health,* the *Yukon Health,* or on the truck or railroad units. We believe their stories are an important part of Alaska's history and should be preserved.

Selected Bibliography

Albrecht, C. Earl. *Public Health Progress in Alaska,* Ketchikan: 1949.

Chevigny, Hector. *Lord of Alaska*. Portland, Oregon: Binford and Mort, 1965.

——. *Russian America*. New York: Ballantine Books, 1965.

Clark, Henry W. *History of Alaska*. New York: The Macmillan Co., 1930.

Devigne, H.C., Dr. *Time of my Life*. New York: Lippincott, 1942.

Emanuel, Richard P. "The Alaska Peninsula." *Alaska Geographic* 21:1 (1994).

Federal Field Committee for Development Planning in Alaska. *Alaska Natives and the Land*. Anchorage: 1968.

Gruening, Ernest. *The State of Alaska*. New York: Random House, 1968.

Kresge, D.T., T.R. Morehouse, and G.W. Rogers. *Issues in Alaska Development*. University of Alaska Institute of Social and Economic Research. Seattle: University of Washington Press, 1977.

Maisel, Albert Q. "Our Neglected Weapon Against Tuberculosis." *Liberty Magazine*. Jan. 11, 1947.

Munoz, Rie. *Nursing in the North*. Juneau: Alaska Nurses Association, 1967.

Patty, S. "Excursion Inlet." *Seattle Times,* Oct. 31, 1976.

——. "Perilous Escape from Siberia." *Seattle Times,* June 20, 1971.

"A Tale of Two Territories" (editorial). *American Journal of Public Health,* July, 1948.